PRAISE FOR *THE YIN YANG DIET*

"Choosing a healthy diet is one of the most important things we can do for our health. Ken Babal's new book cleverly combines recent nutritional science with the traditional Chinese system of yin-yang. He educates us to take nothing in excess but all things in healthy moderation."

— **Mary Hardy, MD**, specialist in botanical and integrative medicine, founder of the Integrative Medicine Clinic at Cedars-Sinai and former Medical Director of the Simms/Mann-UCLA Center for Integrative Oncology

"An interesting book blending western and eastern nutrition making you more aware of what you consume. Delicious and balanced recipes."

— **Thom Tan Nguyen, MD (Vietnam), LAc**, Clinical Supervisor, Emperor's College

"To "eat a balanced diet" is something we've all heard time and time again as a basic dietary guideline. But what is "balanced", exactly? How do we achieve this? What cues should we look for and what are the practical steps to take when embarking on our quest for vibrant health? Ken Babal answers these questions and much more with remarkable insight in *The Yin-Yang Diet*. Homeostasis IS health and Babal nails this critical concept with a fresh, evidence-based take on ancient principles. As dietary trends come and go, this book is an essential and timeless resource to keep on the shelf and refer to over and over."

— **Lawrence Gustafson**, Nutrition Counselor, The Center for Integrative Medicine, Tarzana California

"In *The Yin-Yang Diet*, Ken is able to take a century's old Chinese medicine tradition and apply it to many of the important health questions that we have today in a very accessible way. Applying the information in this book can provide one with a much needed holistic understanding of their body, helping them to find the necessary balance required for both health and healing. These time-proven ancient principles are especially helpful at this critical point in our battle against chronic disease and a medical system that has simply become too costly."

— **Mark J. Kaylor**, Founder, Radiant Health Project

The Yin-Yang Diet

For Balanced Nutrition, Health and Harmony

A Modern Scientific Approach to Balanced Nutrition Based on the Ancient Asian Concept of Yin and Yang

KEN BABAL, CN

The information contained in this book is based upon the research and personal and professional experiences of the author. It is not intended as a substitute for consulting with your physician or other healthcare provider. Any attempt to diagnose and treat an illness should be done under the direction of a healthcare professional.

The publisher does not advocate the use of any particular healthcare protocol but believes the information in this book should be available to the public. The publisher and author are not responsible for any adverse effects or consequences resulting from the use of the suggestions, preparations, or procedures discussed in this book. Should the reader have any questions concerning the appropriateness of any procedures or preparation mentioned, the author and the publisher strongly suggest consulting a professional healthcare advisor.

The Yin-Yang Diet

For Balanced Nutrition, Health and Harmony

KEN BABAL, CN

Turner Publishing Company
Nashville, Tennessee
www.turnerpublishing.com

The Yin Yang Diet: For Balanced Nutrition, Health and Harmony

Cover design: Maddie Cothren
Book design: Tim Holtz

Library of Congress Cataloging-in-Publication Data Upon Request

9781684422555 paperback
9781684422562 hardcover
9781684422579 eBook

Printed in the United States of America

17 18 19 20 10 9 8 7 6 5 4 3 2 1

Contents

Introduction

We are all familiar with the phrase "eat a balanced diet," well-known words of advice, if vague. A friend once defined a balanced meal to me as "a cheeseburger in each hand." According to current government guidelines, eating a balanced diet means choosing foods from each of the five food groups (fruits, vegetables, grains, protein, and dairy) daily.

This is the only dietary advice many people receive from their doctors, though we might consider this progress. The medical establishment has been slow in coming around to nutrition. It wasn't so long ago that doctors used to say that diet has nothing to do with disease except in severe cases of malnourishment, and that taking vitamins will only give you expensive urine. In fact, The American Cancer Society made no recognition of the diet-disease connection until the 1980s. This is tragic when you consider how many lives might have been saved with dietary intervention.

It wasn't until 1988 that the first ever nutrition report by a US surgeon general officially acknowledging the connection between diet and disease was released. In the report, poor nutritional habits were implicated as the main contributors to the leading causes of death, namely heart disease, stroke, atherosclerosis, diabetes, and some forms of cancer. Surgeon General C. Everett Koop stated, "Your choice of diet can influence your long-term health prospects more than any other action you might take."

It was hoped that the surgeon general's report would have the same impact on the public's eating habits as the 1964 government warning about tobacco had on smoking. Unfortunately, the American diet has steadily gotten worse, and infectious and degenerative diseases continue to rise in both young and old people alike.

The death rate from infectious diseases is double what it was in 1980. Cancer rates are increasing. Two-thirds of the population is overweight or obese. Half of those who make it into their 80s are expected to be diagnosed with Alzheimer's disease. Children as young as eight years of age now develop what used to be called "adult-onset diabetes." Seven out of ten Americans take at least one prescription drug. These sad statistics suggest that something is terribly wrong with our diet and lifestyle.

It is generally agreed among dietary experts that if you eat the standard American diet (SAD), you have an increased risk of dying prematurely from cancer, heart disease, or diabetes. What's more, you are more likely to spend your later years in a debilitated condition requiring assistance from family and caregivers. Even if you are fortunate enough to have medical insurance, it may not save you. Reports predict that in the next few years, there will not be enough doctors to care for the growing numbers of sick people.

We witness the SAD in coffee shops, fast-food places, restaurant chains, and supermarkets: double-bacon cheeseburgers, high-sodium frozen meals, and liters of Coke and Pepsi. Noticeably missing from the SAD are vegetables and fruits. A recent survey found that 42 percent of Americans eat fewer han two servings of fruits and vegetables a day. Moreover, the vegetable serving was often French fries or others not associated with reduced disease risk.

Our food is bleached, deodorized, refined, hydrogenated, irradiated, preserved, pasteurized, homogenized, and genetically modified. Food production has moved from a biological process to a chemical manufacturing process (fractionated and restructured). For example, instead of whipped cream, you can find imitation cream whipped topping consisting of hydrogenated oil, high-fructose corn syrup, sodium caseinate, and polysorbate 60 with artificial flavor.

Our modern diet bears little resemblance to that of our ancestors or what humans evolved on. There are glaring nutritional imbalances that need to be corrected if we are to reduce disease occurrence and live up to our full potential. For example, the diet of prehistoric man had about sixteen times more potassium than sodium, whereas modern civilized diets have turned this ratio upside down. Overwhelming evidence suggests that the potassium-sodium imbalance is possibly the single largest contributor to ill health.

Another major imbalance in our modern diet is the ratio of omega-3 to omega-6 fatty acids. Humans evolved and flourished on a high intake of omega-3s from fish, wild game, and plants. Today, the proportion of omega-3 to omega-6 fatty acids has been turned on its head. This fat imbalance has caused us to pay a terrible price: Our blood is too thick, inflammation is out of control, and our brains are literally drying up from a lack of omega-3 fatty acids.

The good news is the human body has an overwhelming tendency to make itself right again. It is an amazing self-repairing machine. The body is constantly renewing itself as old cells are replaced with new copies. Every six months we have new red blood cells. Every five days we have a new stomach lining, and every few years a healthy person has a new skeleton.

We used to think that heart disease was incurable. We now know that the plaque that corrodes arteries is reversible. It is crucial, however, that we provide the body with the required nutrients in the right proportions.

The Chinese have always sought balance in life and in diet. This is what attracted me to traditional Chinese medicine. The Chinese call this balance Yin and Yang. Yin and Yang describe how opposites or contrary forces are interconnected and interdependent. When either Yin or Yang is deficient or excessive (like potassium and sodium), it fails to restrict the other in the balanced relationship between the two.

The Yin-Yang Diet will guide you through the opposing yet complimentary effects of food and nutrients and the biological processes that must be kept in balance in order to prevent disease and achieve vibrant health. I always try to look for universalities in nutrition. When ancient wisdom correlates with modern science, you know you've found truth.

Chapter 1

The Yin-Yang Concept

Life in Balance

Yin-Yang is an ancient Asian concept that describes polar opposites and how they function in relation to each other. It is known as the Great Principle and sometimes referred to as the Law of Opposites. Yin and Yang describe how opposites or contrary forces are interconnected, interdependent, and complimentary. Chinese wisdom suggests that in order to understand anything, we must consider its opposite.

The Yin-Yang concept originated early on, and the terms simply referred to whether or not a place faced the sun. The place that faced the sun or was filled with sunlight was called Yang, while the place that faced away from the sun was called Yin. Later, the ancient Chinese gradually observed that some pairs in the natural world could be similarly objectified, such as heaven and earth, sun and moon, day and night, cold and hot, and so on.

Other easily observed examples of Yin-Yang pairs are male-female, passive-active, masculine-feminine, front and back, and outside-inside. The terms also describe the continuous process of natural change, such as day (Yang) changing into night (Yin) and heat (Yang) alternating with cold (Yin).

Energy moves in a pendulum swing between opposites. Though one may dominate the other, total dominance is not permanent. Eventually, the other takes its turn as the dominant force. One side is neither better nor worse than the other unless it becomes too extreme.

Yin-Yang Pairs

Yang	Yin
Active	Passive
Outside	Inside
Male	Female
Masculine	Feminine
Light	Dark
Heat	Cold
Expansion	Contraction

Yin-Yang Symbol

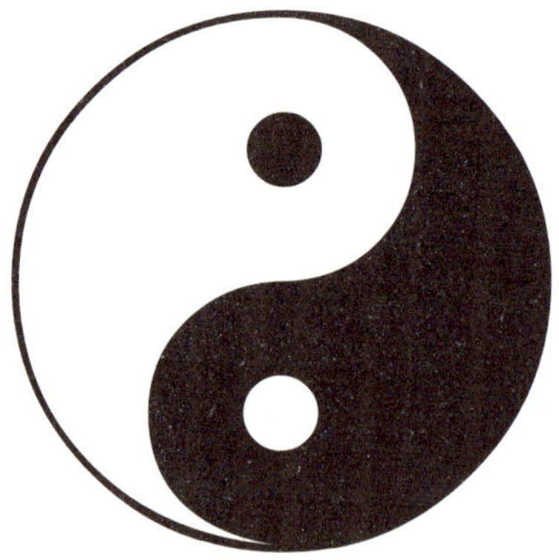

The symbol for Yin and Yang is two interlocking spirals with two dots. Some say it looks like a pair of fishes nestling head to toe. The curve dividing them indicates that Yin and Yang are continuously merging. The symbol illustrates that nothing is purely Yin or purely Yang. It shows Yin within the Yang as the dark eye in the white fish; Yang is shown contained in Yin by the white eye of the dark fish. Everything has both Yin and Yang aspects, though it is either more Yin or more Yang. For example, a peach has soft flesh (Yin) as well as a hard pit (Yang); all males have a female aspect and all females have certain maleness.

It should be pointed out that the Yin-Yang concept is not the same as Western dualism, which sees forces of nature as antagonistic, or as good or bad, or as right or wrong. Eastern dualism sees two forces that antagonize but at the same time are complementary.[1] Lao Tzu, an ancient Chinese philosopher, expressed this complementarity in the Tao Te Ching: "Under heaven, we all know beauty as beauty because there is ugliness. We know virtue because there are bad deeds."

Yin and Yang in Health and Disease

The Yin-Yang principle is the fundamental concept of the traditional Chinese healthcare system, which is more than 3,000 years old and has been practiced on at least a billion people. Yin-Yang theory holds that disease is a result of an imbalance between Yin and Yang. Specifically, it is a hyperactivity or hypoactivity of Yin or Yang. When either Yin or Yang is deficient or excessive, it fails to restrict the other in the balanced relationship between the two. Being too Yin or too Yang without being able to return to balance constitutes a state of disease. In Western terms, dynamic balance is referred to as *homeostasis*.

Illnesses that are characterized by weakness, slowness, coldness, and underactivity are Yin. Illnesses that manifest strength, forceful movements, heat, and overactivity are Yang. Yang symptoms tend to be acute and dramatic but are usually overcome relatively quickly. Yin symptoms, on the other hand, tend to be chronic and more difficult to correct. If disharmony between Yin and Yang is slight, we might feel vaguely off-balance. Though we're not sick, we don't feel exactly well either.

If we wish to maintain equilibrium and stability, it is essential that we understand the principle of Yin and Yang.

Too Much Yin

Appearance—quiet, withdrawn, sluggish, vulnerable, lacks drive; tongue is moist, pale, and slightly swollen.

Traits—weak voice, shallow breathing.

Symptoms—cold, little appetite, frequent urination, clear urine.

Too Much Yang

Appearance—agitated, active, restless; tongue is red and dry.

Traits—loud voice, talkative, heavy breathing.

Symptoms—hot, constipated, dark urine, dry mouth.

Yin and Yang in Diet and Nutrition

In traditional Chinese medicine, food is viewed as medicine, and it is used to nourish and harmonize the body, mind, and spirit. Nutritional balance from a traditional Chinese medicine perspective is much different from that of Western nutrition. Modern nutrition science is based on knowing the chemical composition of foods. Western nutritionists quantify nutrients such as protein, carbohydrates, and fat, then group foods accordingly, with a one-size-fits-all serving recommendation. Chinese nutrition is based on food energetics and the forces of Yin and Yang, and it is applied according to individual needs.

Food heats us or cools us, energizes or calms us, acidifies or alkalizes us. The gentle swing in our metabolism between

Yin and Yang opposites is what keeps us stable. If one side becomes out of proportion for too long, balance is disrupted, we feel unwell, and we become susceptible to disease. If we eat predominantly Yang foods, we become more Yang. If we eat predominantly Yin foods, we become more Yin.

All foods can be classified on a scale as predominantly Yin or Yang. It is a relativity theory based on opposing effects. On the furthest extreme of Yin are fruit, sugar, and alcohol. Eggs, meat, and salt are on the furthest extreme of Yang. Grains, most notably brown rice, are near the middle. This does not mean that foods on the far ends of the scale are bad or that we should eat rice only. It means that extreme foods should be consumed in moderation only by healthy individuals. For example, moderate alcohol (Yin) consumption can have cardiovascular health benefits. But too much can harm the liver and increase cancer risk. Sodium (Yang) is an essential element, but excessive consumption of salt can contribute to high blood pressure. Too much meat (Yang) can cause constipation; too much fruit (Yin) can cause diarrhea; too much in the middle can cause vitamin or mineral deficiencies. We need to strike a balance between Yin and Yang yet be careful to avoid overeating of extreme foods. The majority of one's food intake should consist of non-extreme foods, which have more subtle actions. Swinging from extreme to extreme can keep us balanced, but it is gentler and healthier to maintain balance by moving between less extreme positions.

Yin←Alcohol Sugar Honey Butter Oil Fruit Nuts Tofu Vegetables Seeds Beans Milk Yogurt Cheese (Soft) Sea Vegetables Neutral (Balance Point) Whole Grains Fish Poultry Cheese (Hard) Eggs Red Meat Coffee Salt→Yang

Unlike Western dietary guidelines, the *Yin-Yang Diet* is not a one-size-fits-all approach. Your balance of Yin and Yang foods is determined by your constitution and present condition. A person with a Yang constitution should have a greater proportion of Yin foods in their diet. Conversely, an individual with a Yin constitution can have more Yang foods. Overall, Yang foods are more concentrated and condensed, while Yin foods tend to contain more water.

Yin-Yang theory and how it relates to food was originally imported to the West by George Ohsawa in the 1950s. He termed his system *macrobiotics*, meaning "large or long life." Macrobiotics is defined as a philosophy of living a balanced life, which includes a dietary regimen centered on whole grains and vegetables (both land and sea). According to Ohsawa, healthful eating meant striving for a balance between Yin and Yang.

Like in macrobiotics, the goal of the *Yin-Yang Diet* is Yin-Yang balance. However, it is a modern, scientific approach that is far less restrictive, allowing more variety in food choices. A macrobiotic diet forbids meat, dairy, certain fruits and vegetables, and spices. The *Yin-Yang Diet* does not forbid any food or food group. You can have a little of everything as long as you maintain balance. It's about being flexible, diverse, moderate, and in harmony with your own rhythms and needs.

When you achieve Yin-Yang balance in your diet, you are on the path to what the Chinese call "radiant health" or "health beyond danger." Radiant health is the highest level of health a person can attain.

Chapter 2

Protein and Essential Fatty Acids

Yin-Yang Life Battery

The word "protein" is derived from the Greek *protos,* meaning "first." It is given priority because we are literally made of protein (skin, hair, muscles, organs, tissues, hormones, and so on). The richest sources of protein are meat, fish, poultry, eggs, dairy, beans, nuts, and seeds.

When we digest protein, it is broken down into its component parts, called amino acids, which are then reassembled to build and repair the body's protein structures. Our DNA is actually a blueprint for protein synthesis in the body.

In foods and the human body, protein (Yang) is usually accompanied by fat (Yin). For example, protein and fats are found together in cell membranes and in the lipoproteins that carry fats and cholesterol in the bloodstream.

Fats are comprised of fatty acids, two of which are essential for human health. Like vitamins, they must be supplied by the diet because the body can't make them. Essential fatty acids are components of all cell walls and are required for healthy skin, hair, nails, thyroid and adrenal glands, the nervous system, reproductive function, growth and vitality, oxygen transport, and a healthy cholesterol level.

One of these essential fatty acids (EFAs) is called *linoleic acid* (omega-6 family) and is found primarily in seeds, nuts, and cooking oils (corn, safflower, and sunflower). The other is *alpha-linolenic acid* or simply *linolenic acid* (omega-3 family), found chiefly in flax and chia seeds with small amounts in soybeans, rapeseed (canola), walnuts, and leafy green vegetables. Two fatty acid derivatives of linolenic acid, EPA eicosapentaenoic acid (EPA) and docosahexaenoic acid (DHA), are abundant in oily fish, such as salmon, mackerel, tuna, trout, and sardines. Omega-3 fatty acids are the ones most lacking in our modern diet. (More information in Chapter 3.)

Protein and fats are fundamentally important for the preservation of structure in the living body. As a self-repairing machine, the human body is constantly renewing itself, creating new cells and tissues from protein and fats. The association of fats and protein represent the interaction of Yin and Yang from which energy and life is created—our "life battery," if you will.

Hans Selye, a Canadian scientist who received a Nobel Prize nomination for his work on the nature of stress, observed that every organism has a sort of "life battery" that stores life energy in the same way an electric battery stores electrical current.[1] He wondered what the biochemical basis of this life battery might be and how it might be recharged when run down.

Just like any other battery, your life battery has two poles: a positive and a negative pole between which a current of energy flows. In nutrition terms, protein has a slightly positive charge (Yang), and fats and oils form the negative pole (Yin). Vitamins and minerals keep the current running between the poles. Chinese medicine refers to the energy that flows between them as *chi*, which is renewed on a daily basis.

During conception, protein and fats join to form new life. Sperm, composed largely of protein, fertilizes the ovum, consisting mostly of fat. Note that men have a higher percentage of muscle (protein) whereas women have a higher ratio of fat to muscle.

Yin-Yang Life Battery

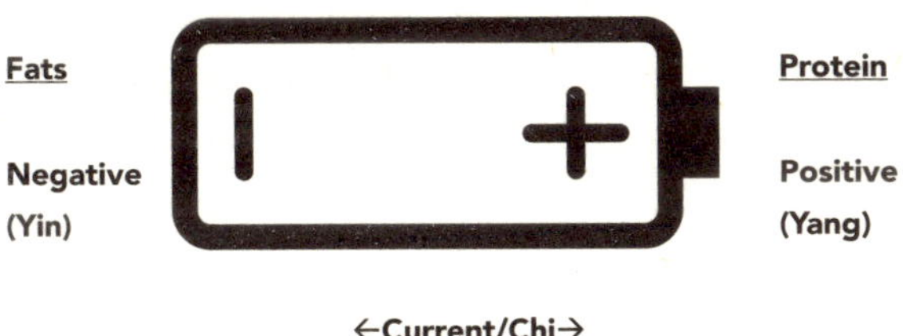

Recharge Your Life Battery

Studies show that many of us don't obtain sufficient amounts of quality protein or EFAs to keep our battery charged. This is often the case with the aged or those who are physically active or experience high stress. Furthermore, many drugs destroy the associations between proteins and fats.

To keep your life battery fully charged, the *Yin-Yang Diet* includes a protein-oil combination of protein powder and flaxseed oil as a shake. Breakfast is an ideal time to consume the shake because it is easily digested and takes little time to prepare. It's a great way to start the day, and it will sustain you until your next meal.

One of the first scientists to consider the health implications of fat consumption was Johanna Budwig, a German biochemist. Dr. Budwig operated a medical clinic in the 1950s and was celebrated for her work with cancer patients. The Budwig protocol included a flaxseed oil–cottage cheese mixture.

Cottage cheese consists of the dairy proteins casein (80 percent) and whey (20 percent), which are rich in the sulfur amino acids cysteine and methionine. Sulfur amino acids make fatty acids more water-soluble and easier to assimilate. Whey is the thin, liquid part of milk remaining after the curds (casein) are removed in cheese making.

Whey, once considered a waste product, is now recognized as a superfood with remarkable applications ranging from protein supplementation to immune support. Most people who are allergic to casein in cow's milk can usually consume whey without problems. Whey protein is low in fat and is easily digested. Whey protein contains small amounts of lactose (much less than is found in milk) but usually too little to cause intestinal problems in those who are mildly lactose-intolerant.

Some people might think of whey protein as a supplement for athletes and body builders. However, whey protein has been shown to reduce muscle wasting in the elderly, reduce risk of diabetes, inhibit cancer development, and defend against cognitive decline.[2]

Whey Protein Benefits

- High biological value (104), utilization, digestibility
- High concentration of amino acids
- Richest source of branched chain amino acids—supports muscle growth
- Richest source of immunoglobulins (protection from infection)—attack foreign tissue
- High in cysteine—supports glutathione production more effectively than free-form cysteine supplements

Yin-Yang Diet Recommendation

Blend one scoop of whey protein with 1 tablespoon of flaxseed oil or an essential oil combination such as Omega Nutrition Essential Balance® in 8 ounces of plant milk (such as soy, rice, hemp, or coconut). If the plant milk is sweetened, dilute it with water.

Variation: Add a half-teaspoon of matcha green tea powder. Green tea is known for its polyphenols, considered to be the best antioxidants in the plant kingdom. Green tea consumption has been associated with a lower risk of heart disease, diabetes, osteoporosis, and certain types of cancer. It protects DNA and has been shown to increase energy expenditure (a benefit for those wishing to lose excess body fat). The modest amount of caffeine in green tea in combination with an amino acid called theanine helps bring about a relaxed state of alertness. Green tea flavor goes well with vanilla-flavored whey protein.

Chapter 3

Fats and Oils

Cardiovascular and Brain Health, Inflammation Control

Our perception and understanding of fats and cholesterol have gone through many changes over the years. Forty years ago, animal fats and cholesterol were vilified. Plant oils and margarine, on the other hand, were promoted as healthful alternatives. Many believed that "fat-free" was the way to go, especially for weight reduction and lowering one's risk of heart disease. The low-fat and fat-free trend had a lot of supporters, but there were glaring inconsistencies and a notable paradox: Why do the French, who consume the most cheese in the world, have lower body weights and a lower rate of heart disease?

It seems the no-fat advocates forgot that some fats are essential. That is, certain fats must be supplied in the diet because the body can't make them. They are required just like vitamins, which is why they used to be called vitamin F. In the case of the French, they have a great appreciation of natural, unprocessed foods and enjoy wine with meals, which counters the saturated fat in cheese by thinning the blood.

Know Your Fats

Asian wisdom tells us that fat consumption supports the Yin principle, is grounding, is warming, and creates a sense of security.

This is why fats are so appealing—we like to feel secure and to slow down and have ample energy and warmth.[1] In foods, they provide much of the pleasing flavor and mouthfeel.

Fat is comprised of fatty acids. Animal foods such as meat and butter contain primarily saturated fatty acids, which are solid at room temperature. Plant foods, cooking oils, and fish contain mostly unsaturated fatty acids, which are liquid at room temperature.

Of the unsaturated fatty acids, two are essential for human health. One is called *linoleic acid* (omega-6 family) found primarily in seeds, nuts, and cooking oils (corn, safflower, and sunflower). The other is *alpha-linolenic acid* or simply *linolenic acid* (omega-3 family) found chiefly in flaxseed and flaxseed oil with small amounts in soybean, rapeseed (canola), walnut, and green leafy vegetables.

EFAs are components of all cell walls and are required for healthy skin, hair and nails, thyroid and adrenal glands, the nervous system, reproductive function, growth and vitality, oxygen transport,and a healthy cholesterol level.

To be healthy, we must maintain balance between animal fats and vegetable fats (oils). By obtaining sufficient amounts of essential unsaturated fatty acids (from fish, plants, and unrefined oils) we are better able to accommodate saturated fats (meat, dairy, butter) in our diet. Too much animal fat in one's diet can crowd out the essential fats and contribute to a high cholesterol level.

Cholesterol is a waxy substance that accompanies fat in animal foods only. Although necessary for health, cholesterol has acquired a bad reputation because it is a component of artery-clogging plaque. Cholesterol is required for producing adrenal and sex hormones, vitamin D, and bile. There is no dietary requirement for cholesterol since the body can make what it needs from saturated fat. In fact, most of the cholesterol in the body is manufactured by the liver and not obtained from food. When dietary cholesterol increases, the body makes less.

Essential, unsaturated fatty acids help keep cholesterol in check by transporting it to the liver for excretion through bile acids. Dietary factors that increase cholesterol production are saturated fats, dietary cholesterol (minimally), trans fats (partially hydrogenated oils), excess refined starches and sugars (which have their vitamins, minerals, and fiber removed), dehydration, and deficiencies of fat-metabolizing nutrients such as choline, inositol, magnesium, zinc, and B-6. Antioxidants, including vitamins A, C, and E, help deter cholesterol deposition in the arteries by preventing harmful oxidation of cholesterol.

Omega-3 to Omega-6 Imbalance

A major imbalance in our modern diet that contributes to much ill health is the ratio of omega-3 to omega-6 fatty acids. Humans evolved and flourished on a high intake of omega-3s from fish, wild game, and plants. Today, the proportion of omega-3 to omega-6 fatty acids has been turned on its head. Typically, the ratio of omega-3 to omega-6 in the American diet is 1 to 10 or 20. Some researchers have suggested that the ideal ratio is 1 part omega-3 to 4 or 5 parts omega-6. Our prehistoric ancestors thrived on a diet with a ratio of about 1:1. The traditional diet that protected Greenland Eskimos from heart attacks, strokes, cancer, and other fat-related diseases was a reverse omega-3 to omega-6 ratio of 2.5: 1. This fat imbalance has caused us to pay a terrible price: Our blood is too thick, inflammation is out of control, and our brains are literally drying up from a lack of omega-3 fatty acids.[2]

The brain is highly sensitive to fats in our diet. The brain is composed of 60 percent fat, especially the omega-3 fatty acid DHA (docosahexaenoic acid), which is found in oily fish along with EPA (eicosapentaenoic acid). The more fish you eat, the more DHA ends up in your brain. Scientific research suggests that a lack of DHA may be a primary cause of many brain disorders on the rise, such as depression, Alzheimer's disease, and attention deficit hyperactivity disorder (ADHD). Autopsies of patients with advanced Alzheimer's disease have shown that their brains had approximately 30 percent less DHA in various areas than the brains of people of the same age without the disease.

One study analyzed the fish-eating patterns of more than 800 men and women (ages 54 to 94) living in nursing homes, then checked for the occurrence of Alzheimer's disease four years later. Researchers found that 131 participants had developed Alzheimer's disease, though frequent fish eaters (those who ate at least one fish meal per week) had a 60 percent lower risk rate than those who never, or hardly ever, ate fish.[3]

An underlying cause of most chronic diseases is inflammation. Normally, when we think of inflammation we think of the "-itis" diseases: arthritis, colitis, gingivitis, and the like, and the characteristic symptoms: pain, redness, and swelling. However, a silent type of chronic, low-grade inflammation also occurs in blood vessels, which has been strongly implicated in heart disease.

Inflammation begins once an artery becomes damaged—for example, from high blood pressure, antioxidant deficiencies, or aging. The injury attracts platelets and white blood cells to repair the damage. These substances promote healing, but they can also cause inflammation and clotting.

The balance of EFAs in your diet is crucial for controlling inflammation. With the help of enzymes, fatty acids are transformed into powerful, hormone-like substances (called eicosanoids) that can ramp up inflammation or tame it down. The eicosanoid derived from linoleic acid (omega-6) constricts blood vessels, increases blood clotting, and can tip the balance toward inflammation. In opposition, the eicosanoid derived from linolenic acid (omega-3) suppresses the inflammatory agents unleashed in the body by an over-abundance of bad omega-6 fats, such as margarine and refined cooking oils. The omega-3 fatty acid EPA competes with arachidonic acid, a pro-inflammatory fatty acid synthesized from linoleic acid. Arachidonic acid is also found in meat, dairy products, and eggs. Too much arachidonic acid leads to platelet aggregation, inflammation, pain, immune suppression, allergies, and skin disorders.

A healthy body can produce EPA and DHA from linolenic acid. DHA is the fatty acid end-product of linolenic acid metabolism and can partially retroconvert to EPA. However, if a person is unhealthy, lacks certain vitamins or minerals, takes medication, or is elderly, he or she may not be able to make the conversions. For this reason, it is advantageous to eat fish, which is a direct source of EPA and DHA.

Many studies show an inverse relationship between fish consumption and heart attack deaths or stroke. As fish consumption increased, the risk of heart disease decreased.

In 1994, The Lyon Diet Heart Study found that a Mediterranean-style diet high in omega-3 fatty acids proved to be more effective in saving lives of heart patients than any drug, lifestyle program, or other diet.[4] Compared to those on the American Heart Association diet, patients on the Mediterranean-style diet experienced an unprecedented 76 percent lower risk of dying from cardiovascular disease, including heart attack and stroke.

To enjoy a high level of health and protection from disease, the omega 3:6 imbalance needs to be corrected. About 85 percent of Americans are deficient in omega-3 fatty acids. Balance can be restored by eating more oily fish, flaxseed, chia seeds, walnuts, and green leafy vegetables and less refined corn, safflower, and sunflower oils. The best oily fish choices (those high in EPA and DHA) are salmon, mackerel, herring, anchovy, sardines, sablefish, and trout. See Appendix 3 for delicious seafood recipes.

Inflammation Fighters

Inflammation fighters include fresh fruit (especially berries, cherries and grapes), leafy vegetables, flaxseed, olive oil, green tea, ginger, garlic, curry and fatty fish.

Good Fats, Bad Fats

Plant oils are extracted from seeds, nuts, and beans. They can be a good source of nutrition or empty calories. The best oils are unrefined. The most common unrefined oils are olive (pressed from the fruit rather than its seed) and flaxseed, which undergo light pressing and filtering to retain their nutrients, color and flavor. Olive oil is prominent in the heart-healthy traditional Mediterranean diet. Most other oils, including corn, soy, sunflower, safflower, and canola (rapeseed) are refined. They are bleached and deodorized and can be identified by their clear color and bland taste. Most of the vitamins, minerals, and some EFA are removed. Processing also introduces toxic molecules that result from the breakdown and alteration of fatty acids. Refined oils are the equivalent of refined (white) flour.

Extra-virgin olive oil is the highest-grade, first pressing of the olive fruit. If it is not labeled as *virgin*, it is refined. Olive, canola, and macadamia oils consists mostly of monounsaturated fatty acids. Monounsaturated fatty acids (omega-9) are not essential but can help lower total cholesterol while increasing HDLs (high-density lipoproteins), the so-called "good cholesterol." The US Department of Agriculture recommends an equal division between saturated, monounsaturated, and EFAs. Flaxseed oil is a refrigerated unrefined oil, and one of the very best sources of omega-3 linolenic acid. It is a fragile oil that is easily destroyed by heat and so should not be used for frying.

Some fats should be avoided at all costs. Rancid (oxidized) fats may be your worst enemy. They contain toxic compounds that impair liver function and are carcinogenic (cancer-causing). Avoid that half-empty, crusty bottle of oil that's been sitting on the table too long at your local diner. Rancid fats can also be found in ground meats and leftovers that have been sitting in the fridge too long. Cheap, rancid oil is frequently used in bottled salad dressings, too, so it's best to make your own. Olive oil will keep for three months unrefrigerated, so buy what you will use in this amount of time.

Check food labels for trans fats. Numerous studies have confirmed that trans fat, a type of unsaturated fat that acts like saturated fat, increases levels of artery-clogging low density lipoprotein (LDL) cholesterol in the blood. Trans fat is formed when food manufacturers combine vegetable oils with hydrogen gas to produce partially hydrogenated oil. This process turns liquid oil into a solid form. Hydrogenated oils are found in margarine and in many packaged snack-food items. Trans fats are foreign to the body, have no function, and interfere with the metabolism of EFAs. They are much worse than cholesterol in raising your blood cholesterol level.

Since 2006, the Food and Drug Administration (FDA) has ruled that packaged foods must list their trans fat content. After 2018, FDA will not allow manufacturers to add artificial trans fats (hydrogenated oil) to food. FDA estimates that the new line on packaged foods' Nutrition Facts Panel and the ban will save many lives by significantly decreasing the number of heart attacks.

Frying is one of the most popular methods of food preparation. It's also the most damaging to your health. High heat causes oils to break down and form toxic chemicals. Antioxidants such as vitamin E and carotene are lost, and EFAs are destroyed. In addition, oxidation of the oil creates unstable molecules (called free radicals) that trigger degeneration of body cells. The result is a toxic stew unfit for human and animal consumption. When medical researchers want to experimentally induce atherosclerosis (artery plaque) in animals, they feed them oil kept at 419 degrees for fifteen minutes. In fast-food restaurants, oils are kept at a high temperature for days.

Brief Asian-style stir-frying is preferable to deep-frying because it uses less oil and a shorter cooking time. When stir-frying, use oil with a higher saturated fat content. Although less beneficial than unsaturated fats, saturated fats stand up to the heat better. Clarified butter (also known as drawn butter or ghee), refined coconut oil, peanut and sesame oils, and olive oil (in that order) are your best choices because they have a higher smoke point. Occasional frying won't kill us, but it can't be recommended for health, especially if trying to reverse a disease. Since high temperatures destroy nutrients, the nutritional benefits of unrefined oils (like olive, flaxseed, and hemp) are best obtained when they are added to food after cooking.

☯ Yin-Yang Diet Recommendation

Reduce your intake of refined safflower, sunflower, and corn oils (cooking oils and many snack items). Instead, favor unrefined oils such as olive and flaxseed. Eat fish (not fried) at least three times per week.

Chapter 4

Carbohydrates: Refined and Unrefined

Glycemic Balance

The three sources of calories are protein, fat, and carbohydrate. Carbohydrate is the body's preferred fuel for energy. If we consume more carbohydrate than what is immediately required for energy, it is stored as body fat. Plant foods are the richest source of carbohydrate—namely grains, legumes, vegetables, and fruits. In their whole, unrefined state, they also provide many vitamins and minerals, fiber, and thousands of important, semi-essential phytonutrients.

Refined carbohydrates are mostly wheat, rice, or corn that has been stripped of its fiber and nutrients and processed into pure starch (white flour and polished rice) or sugar. Foods typically containing white flour and/or sugar are cookies, pies, cakes, candies, pastries, bread, pasta, sugary breakfast cereals, and soda pop.

A hundred years ago, deficiency diseases were discovered in people subsisting on refined flour and polished rice. Today, white flour is "enriched" with a sprinkling of synthetic vitamins to replace what is lost in refining. This raises the question, if someone broke into your home and robbed you of everything you own but then put back a few chairs and a table because they felt sorry for you, would you consider yourself enriched?

If you are so inclined, you can buy back the missing components in the form of a vitamin supplement (for your deficiency) and a fiber supplement (for your constipation).

Whole unrefined carbohydrates are digested and broken down into sugar gradually. Fiber modulates their absorption. Refined carbohydrates, being devoid of fiber, require little digestion and are dumped into the bloodstream quickly. When consumed in a large enough amount, they are a shock to the system and stress our blood sugar control mechanisms.

Insulin is the hormone secreted by the pancreas that lowers the blood sugar (glucose) level by facilitating its entry into muscle cells for energy or to be stored as fat. A spike in the glucose level after consuming a high sugar-load often triggers excess insulin secretion, which can lower the glucose level too far, resulting in hypoglycemia (low blood glucose). Since the brain runs on glucose, a low level can cause us to experience symptoms such as fatigue, irritability, depression, brain fog, or cravings for more sweets or stimulants to raise the blood sugar. This leads to a vicious, addictive cycle. According to a study at Stanford University, approximately 25 percent of Americans are extremely carbohydrate-sensitive and respond with a rapid rise in blood glucose with a corresponding elevation in insulin.[1]

Insulin Resistance and Diabetes

Constant bombardment of cells with alternating high levels of glucose and insulin eventually causes them to lose their sensitivity to insulin (called "insulin resistance"). As a result, glucose and insulin levels remain high, setting the stage for diabetes.

People with Type 1 diabetes produce little or no insulin. In Type 2 diabetes, the pancreas continues to make insulin, but the body is unable to respond to its effects. We used to call Type 2 diabetes "adult-onset diabetes." Today, the term is not used much because children as young as eight years of age are developing Type 2 diabetes. Nearly twenty-five million Americans live with diabetes, and the Centers for Disease Control and Prevention estimate that one in three will have the disease by 2050. The *Wall Street Journal* calls diabetes "a growth industry," because more stores are opening that cater to the needs of the diabetic. It is ironic that diabetes is a leading killer when never before have we known so much about how to prevent and control the disease.

Obesity

An increase in sugars and high-glycemic carbs has fueled the obesity and diabetes pandemic. The new word "diabesity" reflects the tendency for diabetes to be accompanied by obesity. Sharp blood sugar fluctuations lead to insulin resistance and increase the likelihood that calories will be stored as fat. Every successful diet in history has restricted sugar.

Metabolic Syndrome

Insulin resistance, along with abdominal obesity, high blood pressure, high triglycerides, and low HDL (the "good" cholesterol), tend to appear together and are collectively known as syndrome X or metabolic syndrome. Abdominal obesity is defined as a waist circumference of more than 40 inches for men, and more than 35 inches for women. Some doctors make the metabolic syndrome diagnosis if a person has two or more of the conditions.[2] In addition to diabetes, metabolic syndrome increases the risk of heart disease and some types of cancer.

Cancer

Insulin resistance creates an ideal environment for cancer, because tumors need both insulin and high levels of glucose to survive. In this sense, tumors are "sugar-feeders," meaning they are fueled by glucose, not fat or protein. Too much insulin can promote the growth of certain types of cancer, including stomach, colon, endometrial, ovarian, lung, prostate, and breast cancer.[3] In fact, high insulin levels may be the best predictor of whether a woman's breast cancer returns after treatment, since high insulin levels increase the risk of recurrence and death by at least 800 percent. By maintaining a balanced blood sugar level, however, we can selectively starve tumors.

Alzheimer's Disease and Autism

A rapid growth of scientific literature shows a surprising connection between insulin disturbances and other diseases, such as Alzheimer's disease[4] and autism. Mounting evidence implicates diabetes, its predecessor metabolic syndrome, and insulin resistance as important risk factors for Alzheimer's disease. Some researchers are now referring to Alzheimer's disease as Type 3 or brain diabetes, which might be prevented and treated with insulin-sensitizing, anti-diabetes agents.

Insulin's role in cognitive function is becoming more widely accepted, and a recent study suggests a link between autism and diabetes.[5] Both diseases have a common underlying mechanism: impaired glucose tolerance and excess levels of insulin. The problem may begin in the womb, since gestational diabetes is the most important identified maternal risk factor for autism. Based on accumulating scientific evidence, the study's author concludes that insulin needs to be taken seriously as a causative element in autism.

A steady blood sugar level is fundamentally important to healthy functioning of all the body's systems. Disturbed blood sugar levels have profound implications directly related to many functions and conditions, such as energy production, immune function, brain function, mood, menstruation, fertility, aging, and allergies, to name a few.

Health experts warn that most of us are consuming way too much sugar. In 1800, sugar consumption was about 5 pounds per year per person. Today, it is about 160 pounds per year. We are not physiologically equipped to handle such large amounts of sugar. There is nothing inherently wrong with sugar. It's the quantities we consume that are cause for concern. (See Appendix 2 for information on sweeteners.)

Controlling our intake of sugar and high-glycemic foods is the single most important action we can take to improve overall health. Sugar is a delight to the taste buds, and we should enjoy all five flavors every day (sweet, sour, bitter, salty, and pungent). But beware the consequences of excessive intake: tooth decay, blood sugar disturbances, excess acidity, accelerated aging, and mineral depletion.

So, is there a safe sugar dosage? I try to limit sugar to about 15 grams at a time and about one sweet treat per day. This translates to about a half a cup of soda or fruit juice per serving. Just one twelve-ounce can of Coke or Pepsi contains about 39 grams of sugar (more than nine teaspoons). Rather than relying on overly sweet beverages, drink water throughout the day to satisfy your thirst and keep you hydrated.

Keep a diary for a few days to determine how many grams of added sugars you typically consume in a day. Check the Nutrition Facts Panel on packaged foods for the number of grams of added sugar per serving. Multiply by how many servings you consumed, and jot it down. At the end of the day, calculate the total number of grams of sugar you consumed. Keep track of your added sugar intake for three days or more. Do not count sugars from whole foods such as vegetables and fruits. If a packaged food has added sugar, it will appear in the ingredient listing as sugar, sucrose, fructose, or similar.

Examples of Packaged Foods that Typically Contain Added Sugars

Ketchup	Jam	Desserts
Candy	Sodas	Canned fruits
Cereals	Fruit juices	
Cookies	Snack foods	

The American Heart Association suggests no more than 25 grams per day of added sugars for women, and 37.5 grams for men. A teaspoon of sugar is 4 grams. Don't feel guilty if you occasionally slip up. Nobody is going to criticize you for having a piece of cake on your birthday. It's not what you do on occasion that matters but what you do as a routine. Sometimes it is unavoidable. If you know you'll be having a high-glycemic meal (a Sunday morning Boy Scout pancake breakfast, for example), take a fiber supplement prior to the meal to modulate its effects.

There is one exception when it is acceptable and even recommended to ingest a larger amount of sugar (about 30 grams or more). This is after intense physical activity when muscle cells are screaming for sugar. This is a critical time of increased insulin sensitivity. Satisfying this demand for sugar will rapidly restore muscle glycogen (stored sugar) needed for recovery.

Yin-Yang Diet Recommendation

Reduce your consumption of sugar and other refined carbs. If you crave sweets, it usually means one of two things: You've gone too long without eating a meal, or you didn't balance your meal in Yin and Yang.

Top Ten Foods for a Healthy Blood Sugar Level

1. Oats
2. Soy
3. Cinnamon
4. Bitter melon
5. Mushrooms (*Agaricus* and maitake)
6. Pomegranate
7. Pumpkin
8. Seaweed
9. Leafy greens
10. Fish

Sugar Blues

(Effects of Excessive Sugar Consumption)

1. Rots teeth
2. Food for bacteria, yeasts, fungi, and cancer cells
3. Increases triglycerides (a blood fat)
4. Interferes with vitamin C transport (compromises immune function)
5. Can increase adrenaline production by up to 4 times (a stressor)
6. Contributes to cross-linking of proteins (speeds aging)
7. Removes calcium, magnesium, chromium, and other minerals from the body

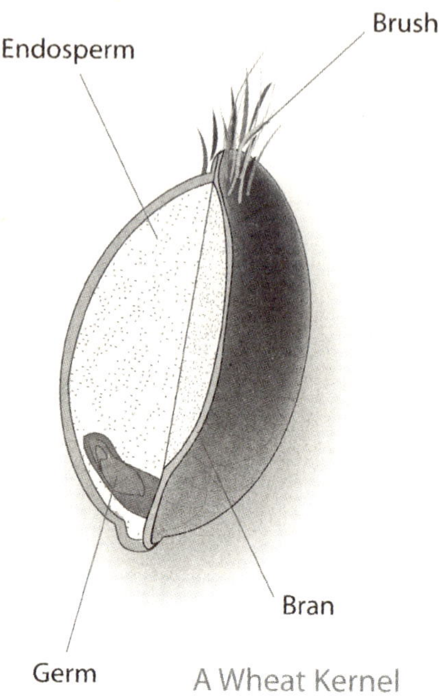

A Wheat Kernel

Grain Anatomy

The structure of whole grains can be separated into three parts: germ, endosperm and bran.

Germ—The germ is the reproductive part of the grain that germinates to grow into a plant. The germ is retained as an integral part of whole-grain foods. It is a rich source of vitamin E and unsaturated fatty acids, which have a tendency to oxidize and become rancid in storage. Thus, germ removal improves the storage qualities of flour. Wheat germ is sold as a popular health food.

Endosperm—The endosperm constitutes the largest part of the grain and is composed chiefly of starch. Refining of grains is intended to isolate the endosperm, which is ground into flour. The rest of the grain is included in whole wheat flour.

Bran—The bran portion is the covering. Bran is particularly rich in dietary fiber. Removal of bran produces flour with a white rather than a brown color. Wheat bran is sold as a fiber supplement and remedy for constipation.

Chapter 5

Sodium and Potassium

A Balancing Act

As astronomer Carl Sagan once noted, minerals are our link to the universe. We are literally composed of the same chemical elements that were once part of a star. Sodium is the sixth most abundant element in the Earth's crust. Table salt is comprised of sodium and chloride, and its chemical formula, NaCl, is familiar to many people. Potassium, an element which takes the symbol K, was first isolated from potash, the ashes of plants, which is how its name is derived.

Sodium, which occurs in all foods, is essential for health and dangerous in excess. Sodium deficiencies, although rare, can be caused by excessive sweating, vomiting or diarrhea. Symptoms include weight loss, weakness, and muscle cramping.

When people think of sodium and health, most think of blood pressure. The common perception is if you have high blood pressure, you must decrease sodium in your diet. But people assume if you are not salt-sensitive, sodium is not an issue, and you can eat all the potato chips and French fries you like.[1]

Actually, nothing is further from the truth. To be healthy, all of us should limit sodium intake while keeping potassium high. The ratio of these two minerals affects every cell in the body. In a sort of see-saw balance, potassium (Yin) helps keep sodium (Yang) in check. So, even if your blood pressure doesn't rise with salty foods, you are still putting yourself at risk for certain diseases if sodium and potassium are out of balance. It's a classic example of Yin-Yang interplay.

There is overwhelming evidence that a dietary excess of salt coupled with a lack of potassium is possibly the single largest contributor to ill health in the United States. In addition to heart attack, stroke and hypertension, one's dietary potassium-to-sodium ratio is believed to be a factor in osteoporosis, asthma, ulcers, stomach cancer, cataracts, kidney stones, and possibly other diseases that appear unrelated. The good news is that by increasing potassium in your diet (vegetables and fruits) and decreasing salt intake, you are creating a healthier balance that can lower your risk of a dozen or so diseases.

Sodium used to be scarce. For most of human history, salt was so scarce the human body learned how to hoard it. Through the millennia, kidney cells developed mechanisms to tenaciously hang on to sodium, returning it back to the bloodstream while squandering potassium.

The diet of prehistoric man had about sixteen times more potassium than sodium, whereas modern civilized diets have turned this ratio upside down. Today, the average American diet contains about 1.6 times more sodium than potassium. This is because we eat more than a week's worth of salt every day while eating only two-thirds as much potassium as we should.

Today, our diets consist largely of processed foods instead of fresh whole foods. Food refining and processing reduces potassium. For example, three-fourths of the potassium in polished (white) rice and white flour disappears. To compound the problem, salt is added to most packaged foods to compensate for the lack of fresh flavor and to satisfy our craving for salt. Since salt alkalizes the system, it is often craved by people who are overly acidic.

The Sodium-Potassium Pump

The sodium-to-potassium ratio is often called "the vitality ratio," and for good reason. In the body's cells, sodium and potassium, assisted by the energy currency adenosine triphosphate (ATP), act as a pump to move compounds through cell membranes. This is commonly called the "sodium-potassium pump," and it is a component of almost all animals—even one-celled organisms. The pumps are actually proteins in cell membranes that pull potassium into the cell interiors and push sodium out. In the process, they generate a voltage between the inside and outside of the cell similar to that of a battery. This "battery" drives electrical signals along nerves and determines the tension and relaxation of muscle cells. It also enables glucose to enter cells and to become fuel for the energy of the cell to perform all its functions. If the potassium-to-sodium balance is not right, the battery doesn't become fully charged, and cell membranes function as if they were old. This imbalance also results in calcium being forced out of cells. For this reason, some researchers believe that a high-salt diet is a greater hazard for osteoporosis than a low-calcium diet. The more salt one eats, the more calcium the body loses in urine, creating more opportunity for calcium kidney stones to form.

The energy used by all these tiny sodium-potassium pumps amounts to about one-fourth of all the calories consumed by people in caloric balance. The body wouldn't expend this much energy on one function unless there was a very important reason.

Salt Has Many Powers

Salt is on the extreme end of Yang, so it must be used with caution, particularly by those with a Yang constitution. Sodium attracts water, and too much causes tissues to retain water, putting pressure on blood vessel walls and dangerously increasing blood pressure. Kidneys purify and recycle body water. Their fragile blood vessels are very sensitive to high blood pressure and can become damaged.

We witness salt's effect in food preparation. Salt tends to dehydrate foods, such as when added to cooking water to keep vegetables and pasta firm. In food preservation, salt draws out moisture, discouraging bacteria, which thrive in moisture.

Because of its extreme Yang nature, salt can be used as a medicine for a temporary quick fix. For example, when blood pressure is too low due to adrenal exhaustion, increasing salt intake can boost blood pressure, alleviating light-headedness and weakness. Also, when the pH of the body becomes extremely acidic, a half-teaspoon of baking soda (sodium bicarbonate) in half a glass of water between meals will produce a noticeable elevation of pH (toward alkalinity) rather quickly. Because of their potentially medicinal effects, extreme Yin or Yang foods sometimes account for conflicting studies and headlines that confuse consumers.

Confusing Headlines

Scientists say that salt, once thought good for you, then bad, then good, then bad, then good again, now definitely bad

Bill Maher

Sodium Requirements

Under the Food and Drug Administration's food labeling rules, the Daily Value for sodium is 2,400 milligrams. (One teaspoon of salt contains about 2,000 milligrams sodium.) However, a human adult can maintain sodium balance with intakes of fewer than 200 milligrams per day, excluding losses due to excessive sweating.

Unfortunately, due to the vast consumption of processed foods and highly salted restaurant meals, the average American ingests three to seven grams (3,000 to 7,000 milligrams) of sodium per day. Processed food accounts for up to 75 percent of the salt intake in a typical American diet. Only about 10-15 percent comes from the salt shaker. Canned vegetables and soups, pickles, and snack foods are usually very high in sodium. Half a can of soup contains, on average, 1,000 milligrams of sodium, nearly half the normal quota for an entire day. A large frozen dinner can contain a whopping 5,000 milligrams! Fast foods are notoriously high in sodium. A quarter-pounder cheeseburger with fries and a shake contains about 1,600 milligrams of sodium (equal to two-thirds of a teaspoon of salt). Cured meats, such as sausage, salami, ham, bacon, hot dogs, and corned beef are reservoirs of sodium, and some fish products, such as smoked salmon and anchovies, contain more salt than the seawater they came from.

How to Improve the Potassium-to-Sodium Ratio

When you eat whole, unprocessed foods, you are going to get very little sodium and large amounts of potassium. Most fruits, vegetables, and legumes (beans, peas, and lentils) are loaded with potassium with little sodium. Even though ocean fish live in a high-salt environment, they still have three to five times as much potassium in their flesh as sodium. The DASH (Dietary Approach to Stop Hypertension) diet often recommended for hypertension emphasizes fresh fruit and vegetables. Ironically, when doctors prescribe diuretics to treat hypertension, they are depleting the body of potassium.

Ethnic groups that do not add common salt to their food have lifelong low blood pressure. So, use salt modestly, and when you do, use unrefined sun-evaporated sea salt, called Celtic grey salt. Celtic salt contains 82 trace minerals in addition to sodium chloride. Common refined sea salt is stripped of its minerals. Of the various types of salt, unrefined sea salt is the most balanced.

In Finland, educating people about eating high-potassium foods and keeping salt consumption down along with the use of a salt substitute (potassium chloride) resulted in lower blood pressure and an astonishing 60 percent drop over twenty years in premature deaths from stroke and heart disease.[2] This proves that small dietary sacrifices can provide rewarding health benefits.

Some High-Potassium Foods

Food	Serving	Potassium (mg)
Beet greens (boiled, drained)	1 cup	1309
White beans (canned)	1 cup	1189
Tomato products, canned, puree	1 cup	1098
Potato, baked with skin	1 medium	926
Plums, dried (prunes)	½ cup	637
Raisins	½ cup	598
Lima beans, cooked	½ cup	485
Banana	1 medium	422
Spinach, cooked	½ cup	420
Artichoke, cooked	1 medium	343
Tomato	1 medium	292
Orange	1 medium	237
Almonds	1 ounce	200

For more information, search the USDA food composition database.

The Food and Nutrition Board of the Institute of Medicine has established an adequate intake level of potassium at 4,700 mg/day for adults.

Yin-Yang Diet Recommendation

The potassium-sodium ratio is the most important mineral ratio in our diet and in the body. Keep it in balance by avoiding high-sodium processed foods and making sure you consume generous amounts of vegetables at most meals. If desired, season foods with modest amounts of Celtic grey salt, Lite salt, or a salt substitute.

Caution: Some people may need to restrict potassium intake for medical reasons. Those with kidney disease are not able to properly excrete potassium.

A Prized Commodity

Salt has been a prized commodity for centuries. The expressions "salt of the earth" and "worth his weight in salt" reflect the high value historically placed on this abundant mineral as a nutrient, seasoning, preservative and medicinal. Roman soldiers were paid in salt, and the word "salary" is derived from sal, the Latin word for salt.

Chapter 6

Digestion and Elimination

Nourish and Cleanse

Weight problems, eczema, acne, allergies, asthma, fatigue, constipation, anemia, gall stones, insomnia, infections, fungal problems, arthritis, osteoporosis, and certain types of cancer: What do these ailments have in common? All can be caused or worsened by poor digestion. Fact is, digestion is a key issue in any type of health problem and one of the most important factors influencing one's total well-being.[1]

As a nutritionist, I know that if I can help a client resolve difficulties with digestion and elimination, we've achieved a great advantage in overcoming other health problems, whether minor or severe. When a person maintains efficient digestion, a strong body chemistry results, and all other systems benefit. Also, if your digestion is functioning properly, you have a better chance of maintaining well-being.

Digestion is a critical facet of nutrition. Nutrition is not just what we eat but what the cells of the body actually receive—and the cells only receive what is broken down through the process of digestion. Nutrients must traverse membrane barriers on a long voyage from the digestive tract into and out of the cells of the intestinal mucosa, vascular system, and finally, the cell membrane. What the cells actually receive is rarely, if ever, optimum. To rephrase an old adage, we are not what we eat but what we digest and absorb.

The flip side of nutrient availability/absorption is how well we get rid of the waste products. Cleansing and nourishing are the two factors in the health equation. Both processes occur within the gastrointestinal tract, which is our fueling station as well as our waste-management system.

Digestive disturbances are very common, and it is safe to say that most people experience some difficulty, especially those who do not enjoy good health. The prevalence of advertisements for antacids alone testifies to the extent of the problem. Stomach acid blockers are among the best-selling drugs of all time. Many of us accept indigestion as a normal part of eating, when in fact we should be barely conscious of digestion. Gas, heartburn, bloating, burping, bad breath, constipation, diarrhea, and general discomfort or fatigue after meals are common symptoms of poor digestion. Although common, these symptoms should not be considered normal. They are distress signals that tell us the process is not going smoothly and we are not getting the full benefit of what we ate. They are also a warning that more serious problems may be down the road if we do not make the necessary dietary changes that prevent these occurrences. Big problems always start small, and minor digestive disturbances can eventually lead to ulcers or conditions affecting other body systems not commonly associated with the gastrointestinal tract.

When things go wrong in the intestinal tract, foreign substances normally excluded, such as toxins, partially-digested food, and microorganisms, are absorbed and distributed throughout the system. This increased permeability of the intestinal mucosa, or "leaky gut" as it is sometimes called, is suspected of contributing to a number of systemic disorders including allergies, eczema, hives, autoimmune diseases, bowel diseases, and viral and bacteria infections. Sometimes the body can go for years with dietary abuse and faulty digestion with little overt sign of problems developing below. By the time they manifest, the connection is often missed.

The good news is that cells of the gastrointestinal lining turn over rapidly, and healthy new cells are constantly replacing old, worn-out ones. Remarkably, every five days you have a new stomach lining. This means that if you are kind to your stomach and balance your food intake according to your constitution and condition, you can expect noticeable improvements in digestion and well-being in just a matter of days. You will then be on the road to radiant health.

Western Medical Approach

The Western medical approach to stomach problems is often a prescription for a stomach acid blocker (proton pump inhibitor), and the patient is allowed to go on eating in their usual unhealthy fashion. The doctor's concern is that unchecked inflammation and irritation in the stomach and esophagus can lead to more serious conditions, including cancer. Esophageal cancer is increasing dramatically, particularly in men 30 to 50 years of age.[2]

Stomach acid blockers help alleviate symptoms of stomach distress such as heartburn or acid reflux, but continued use can cause vitamin B12 deficiency and increase the risk of intestinal infections, bone loss, and dementia.[3,4] These drugs were never intended to be used long-term. Normally, the stomach is an acid environment and needs to be acid in order to inhibit bacteria and assimilate nutrients. In fact, too much stomach acid is often not the problem. Often, it is a *lack* of stomach acid. This might sound contradictory, but think of it this way: If we don't secrete enough stomach acid, food sits in the stomach too long and can cause undesirable fermentation or "bad" acids. Furthermore, we might experience a delayed secretion of our "good"stomach acid, adding to the overall acid load. This is why some people find that taking a little apple cider vinegar in water at mealtimes actually helps prevent acid indigestion.

One might counter that if the drug alleviates symptoms, it is proof that a person produces too much stomach acid. However, if the integrity of the stomach lining is compromised, any amount of stomach acid, even a small amount, can cause irritation.[5] In this case, we might use soothing herbs and foods, such as aloe vera and licorice, which protect the stomach lining and allow it to heal. Most natural practitioners recommend a form of licorice called deglycrrhizinated licorice (DGL). Since glycyrrhizin in licorice can temporarily elevate blood pressure, the glycyrrizin component has been removed. *As a precaution, if you are currently taking prescription acid blockers, work with your doctor to determine when it would be appropriate to come off them.*

Digestion and Traditional Chinese Medicine

Famous for its use of metaphor, traditional Chinese medicine (TCM) views digestion as a liquid, bubbling cauldron with a hot flame (called *digestive fire*) burning beneath it. The stomach is the cauldron where food is broken down into its elements. Digestive fire is the energy (chi) provided by glands and organs for the process to occur. When digestive fire is strong and the mix in the pot is balanced in Yin and Yang, digestion proceeds smoothly and impurities are separated out. Too much cold can compromise digestive function and impair nutrient assimilation. In contrast, too much heat can cause an increased rate of digestion and excessive hunger.

The stomach is said to like moisture and dislike dryness. That's why having some warm broth or tea with a meal helps to stimulate digestive secretions. However, too much liquid (particularly cold beverages) can dilute stomach secretions and cause fats to congeal.

Extreme moisture (Yin) or dryness (Yang) is not good for digestion or overall health. Too much moisture dampens the digestive flame and contributes to obesity, yeast overgrowth, cysts, tumors, abdominal bloating, water retention, and a feeling of stomach heaviness. Besides drinking too much liquid with meals, other habits that contribute to excessive dampness are eating too much cold food, dairy, raw fruit, or salads. To balance excessive dampness, favor warm or cooked foods and warming herbs and spices such as ginger, clove, cinnamon, garlic, and hot peppers (in moderation).

Too much dryness or heat can be troublesome as well. It is often brought on by mental stress and overwork as well as too much red meat, coffee, spicy foods, and overeating. This condition is characterized by a burning sensation in the stomach, stomach ulcers, canker sores, and constipation. Emphasize liquids (mostly between meals), chamomile tea, and relatively more raw food and juices. Cabbage juice has been a longstanding remedy for ulcers (½ cup, three times per day before meals).

Constipation

Constipation is a decrease in the frequency of bowel movements accompanied by a difficult, prolonged effort in passing a hard stool. All too often doctors casually shrug off this condition, saying that it is completely normal for some people to only have two or three bowel movements per week.

Natural health practitioners tend to view this as incorrect and dangerous advice. Normally, it takes up to twenty hours for food to move through the digestive tract. Ideally, it should take twelve to eighteen hours. Also, if you are straining or have any discomfort during elimination, you are probably constipated.

The most common cause of constipation is a lack of fiber in the diet. However, other factors can contribute, such as certain drugs, some iron or calcium supplements, or hypothyroidism. For most people, increasing fiber and liquids solves the problem. Physical activity is also very helpful. Reliance on stimulating laxatives causes dependency and loss of natural function.

Diarrhea

Diarrhea is an abnormally frequent passage of loose, watery stools. It's the body's way of getting rid of something it can't use. Often, diarrhea is caused by a bacterial infection such as food poisoning. Dietary diarrhea can be caused by certain foods such as citrus juice, figs, prunes, coffee, or unripe fruit. Generally, loose stools are unabsorbed food caused by weak digestion or an imbalance of one's food selections. The non-digestible sugar alcohols sorbitol, mannitol, and xylitol used as sugar substitutes in candies and gum can cause diarrhea, gas, and bloating when consumed to excess.

Some natural remedies for diarrhea are blackberry tea, carob powder, and a BRAT diet (banana, white rice, peeled apple, and white toast). Other remedies are activated charcoal, bismuth, and psyllium seed powder (which creates bulk and helps to form a stool). Natural infection fighters for managing diarrhea caused by bacteria are goldenseal and *Citricidal* (grapefruit seed extract). All antibiotic treatments, whether natural or prescription, should be followed with probiotic supplementation. Probiotics help maintain a favorable balance of intestinal flora. Diarrhea, when not caused by a serious disorder, can usually be cured by taking one teaspoon of apple cider vinegar in water with meals and several times a day between meals.

For persistent diarrhea, be sure to consult a physician. Chronic diarrhea can be a symptom of a more serious condition such as parasitic infection or inflammatory bowel disease, and it can be life-threatening in children or the elderly by causing dehydration and loss of electrolyte minerals.

☯ Yin-Yang Diet Recommendations

Do not over-eat. Smaller more frequent meals are best.

You are less likely to tax your digestive capability when you eat modestly—and you'll be able to eat again sooner! Divide your food intake into three meals per day plus one or two snacks. Another benefit: Calories are less likely to be stored as fat when spaced throughout the day.

Keep meals simple and as nutritious as possible.

For easiest digestion, combine only protein + vegetable or grain + vegetable or eat a "mono meal " (a meal of only a single food).

Keep sweets to a minimum.

Sugars tend to ferment in the warm environment of the stomach. Excessive amounts can cause gas, bloating and indigestion. ("Things sweet to taste prove in digestion sour."—Shakespeare)

Eat regular meals but only when truly hungry.
If you experience digestive discomfort, do not eat again until you feel completely comfortable with your last meal.

Do not consume ice-cold or sugary drinks with meals.
Drink only unchilled water, diluted juice, or tea. Icy cold drinks may be appropriate on a hot day, but they can also be a shock to the system and cause fats to congeal in the stomach. Digestive herb teas are especially good to sip with or after meals. Liquids activate digestive juices, but excessive amounts can also dilute them.

Relax—do not eat hurriedly.
Chew food well, and don't eat a lot when feeling nervous or anxious. Stress causes the digestive system to shut down. It's only natural to eat until we're full. However, if we eat hurriedly, we don't give the brain a chance to receive the signal that we're satisfied, and we tend to overeat.

Obtain plenty of fiber in the diet.
Fiber is found in unrefined plant foods (whole grains, beans, vegetables, and fruits). Fiber works like a broom for the intestine, sweeping it clean. However, patients with acute bowel inflammation may need to temporarily reduce their fiber intake. Breads and cereals should provide at least three grams of fiber per serving.

Limit or eliminate coffee (regular and decaf), alcohol, and all drugs not prescribed by your doctor as they can irritate the stomach lining.

Mindful Eating in a Fast Food World

In today's fast-paced world, we're often distracted and don't pay much attention to what we're eating, how we're eating, or how our food choices affect us or the planet for that matter. We might call this mindless eating. The opposite is mindful eating. Mindful eating is a slower, more thoughtful way of eating. You are eating with the intention of caring for yourself and with the attention necessary to enjoy your food and its beneficial effects.

A cornerstone of mindful eating is to slow down. It's not unusual for customers at a fast food place to finish a meal in ten minutes while standing. Most fast foods can be eaten while steering a car, and the restaurants are usually drive-through.

Research has shown that overweight men and women take in fewer calories when they slow their eating pace. A recent Japanese study involving 1,700 young women concluded that eating more slowly resulted in feeling full sooner and eating fewer calories. Eating slowly and mindfully not only helps you eat less, it enhances the pleasure of the dining experience. Wait a few minutes before going for seconds, because it takes a while for the brain to get the message that you're full.

In a world of impulsive choices and immediate gratification, it helps to take a moment to ask yourself a few questions before eating: What did I have at my last meal? Have I had any vegetables and fruits today? Am I truly hungry? If you've experienced digestive discomfort, don't eat again until you are completely comfortable with your last meal. Express gratitude by saying a prayer or thanking the fish that gave its life for your nourishment.

There's no denying that eating the standard American diet (SAD) results in an increased risk of dying prematurely from cancer, heart disease, or diabetes. So, it's good to have a plan and practice mindful eating. But don't stress over food. That can't be good either.

Fiber: The Superstar Non-Nutrient

Grandmother called it roughage. It's also called "the essential non-digestible" and "the indigestible indispensable." Dietary fiber is technically not a nutrient, because it is not broken down and assimilated by the body. We derive no calories or energy from it even though it's classified as a carbohydrate. Nevertheless, fiber is crucial for regulating digestion and may help prevent many diseases, including diabetes, obesity, heart disease, and cancer.

Fiber is essential for a healthy gastrointestinal tract. It exercises the colon by stimulating contractions of the intestine, and works like a broom, sweeping it clean. Fiber also helps to hold moisture in the colon and loosen and soften debris that might otherwise become trapped. Yet another benefit is its ability to act like a sponge, absorbing fats and carbs and slowing their entry into the bloodstream.

Fiber also transports cholesterol and toxins out of the body via bile excretion. Cholesterol reduction has the benefit for lowering heart disease risk. Fiber might also reduce high blood pressure. For diabetics, viscous fiber found in beans and oats slows absorption of carbs and can normalize blood sugar and insulin response. Also, there is evidence that higher fiber intakes can help prevent weight gain or promote weight loss by extending the feeling of fullness after a meal.

The best sources of fiber are unrefined plant foods: fruits, vegetables, beans, and particularly whole grains. We need about 25 to 35 grams of dietary fiber a day. However, when a person is unwilling or unable to make the necessary changes in the diet, a fiber supplement becomes necessary. There are some caveats, though. Although most of us can benefit from increasing fiber, too much of a good thing can create problems. Many people take fiber supplements to prevent constipation. However, taking too much too soon can bind you, causing gas and bloating. I suggest starting with less than the label dosage, then gradually increasing it daily to the point where elimination responds favorably. Be sure to take it with adequate fluid and take it on an empty stomach or before eating.

Chapter 7

Food and Food Abstinence

Immunity, Longevity and Weight Control

Just as the body requires sleep and wakefulness, movement and rest, it also requires food and food abstinence. If you've been neglecting your health by eating poorly or over-indulging, you might benefit from a fast. A fast can be an excellent way to make a fresh start and correct dietary abuses that can show up in the form of lowered immunity, fatigue, allergic reactions, or worsening of chronic conditions. Fasting can desensitize the body to food allergens, permit toxins and debris to be cleared from the liver and kidneys, normalize digestive function, and promote health in general. During a fast, the process of eliminating dead and dying cells is accelerated, as is the development of new cells.

Fasting is one of the oldest therapeutic methods known to man. Nearly all cultures and religions of the world use fasting as a means of improving health or spirituality. Various forms of fasting were employed by Jesus, Muhammad, Buddha, and Gandhi.

A common misconception about fasting is that it is starvation. Starvation, however, is an involuntary weakening and wasting of the body from an extreme and prolonged lack of food, whereas fasting is a voluntary process that has a beginning and an end with health benefits. A fast gives the body a physiological rest. More importantly, it is a decisive step toward taking control over one's health. Fasting does not necessarily require staying home in bed or curtailing activities. A person can usually engage in all non-rigorous daily activities he or she normally would (except eating, of course.)

The delicate relationship of food and health is often evident during a fast. Symptoms of food allergy/hypersensitivity generally lessen or disappear altogether. For example, people who react to the nightshade family of plants (tomato, potato, eggplant, peppers) with joint inflammation and pain invariably experience relief from their symptoms when these foods are withdrawn. Others have attained remissions from various diseases through regular fasting. We know that some animals with certain kinds of illnesses instinctively stop eating. Digestion is an energy-consuming process, and when food is abstained from, the body may be able to concentrate its energy toward fighting the illness. Furthermore, in healthy individuals, fasting triggers the release of hormones that stimulate the immune system.

Caloric Restriction

Restricting calories is a scientifically proven technique known to consistently extend the life expectancy of animals. Undernutrition, as it is sometimes called, has increased the life expectancy of some species by as much as two to three times and has worked in every species tested. Undernutrition should not be confused with malnutrition. In an undernutrition regimen, the total calorie intake is limited, but there is no lack of essential nutrients.

Intermittent fasting, with no restriction on the eating days except that the food be highly nutritious, has also been shown to extend lifespan. As early as the 1940s, researchers studied the effects of intermittent fasting on the lifespan of rats. Rats were fed a high-quality diet and as much as they wanted during eating days but were fasted every second day. Other groups of rats in the study were fasted respectively, either every second, third, or fourth day. The maximum life span of animals that did not fast at all was 800 days but in the fasted groups it was 1,000 to 1,100 days, a 20 to 30 percent extension of maximum life span.[1] Since that time, hundreds of studies have looked at the effects of caloric restriction, with the bulk of them reflecting similar findings.

Caloric undernutrition has other benefits, too. Cancers, cataracts, discoloration and matting of hair, dryness of skin, kidney disease,and heart disease are all less frequent in restricted animals than in normal ones, according to Roy Walford, M.D.[2]

Walford was a life extension researcher at University of California, Los Angeles, School of Medicine, who recommended a regimen of total abstinence from food two successive days each week and a healthful, supplemented diet the other five days. He found this approach easier than eating a low-calorie diet seven days a week.

Types of Fasts

There are several different healthy ways of fasting. The most common way to fast is from early in the evening until you "break-fast" the following morning. Many of us are eating all the way up to bedtime, and the digestive organs don't have a chance to rest.

A modified juice fast, however, from three to five days in duration, is a quick way to get back on tract, let the body "catch up" on its duties, and move toward a higher level of wellness. In a modified juice fast, no solid food is taken, only liquids such as diluted fruit juice, herb teas, vegetable juice and broth, and distilled water. Total intake of fluids should be 1 ½ to 2 quarts per day, an amount normally obtained from foods when eating.

Some practitioners feel that diluted fruit juices and/or lemon water are particularly useful early in a fast because of their cleansing properties. Vegetable juices, on the other hand, are viewed by some as rejuvenating and are favored in the latter stages of the fast. Fresh, raw juices or lactic acid-fermented juices with their active enzymes are preferred over the typical canned/bottled varieties. Sweet vegetable juices such as carrot and beet should only be taken a quarter to half-cup at a time or diluted with a green juice such as celery to avoid stressing the body's blood sugar control mechanisms.

Good choices for fasting herb teas are red clover, chaparral, pau d'arco, burdock root, comfrey, *Echinacea*, fenugreek, and dandelion, but any favorite may be used. They can be drunk warm, cool, or at room temperature.

The type of fasting that is trending now is intermittent fasting (called the 5:2 diet), which entails restricting food intake on two days per week while eating normally on the other days. Typically, on fasting days a person will consume 500 to 600 calories or about 30 percent of what they would normally eat, from two highly nutritious meals. Research shows that calorie restriction from this type of partial fast can help maintain a healthy weight.

Studies have compared the 5:2 diet with calorie cutting on a daily basis.[3,4] In one study, researchers divided 166 overweight middle-aged women into two groups. Both were told to cut calories by 25 percent—one by trimming the calories in each meal, the other by following a 5:2 plan. The women were told to eat a high-protein Mediterranean-style diet of vegetables, fruits, whole grains, nuts, seafood, and olive oil with only moderate amounts of dairy, poultry, eggs,and lean meat. After six months, both groups lost about the same weight. However, those in the 5:2 group experienced more of a decline in insulin resistance (improved blood sugar control) than those who cut calories daily. Moreover, in a three-month trial, women on the 5:2 diet lost more body fat. Why did the 5:2 dieters do better? They were more likely to stick to their plan.

Detoxification Aids

Products that help with cleansing and detoxification are of great benefit during a fast. They include fiber supplements such as psyllium seed powder. Psyllium seed is a soluble fiber that holds moisture in the colon and helps loosen and soften debris that may become trapped in pockets of the intestines. One teaspoon of the whole seed powder or one tablespoon of husks is added to eight ounces or more of water or diluted fruit juice. The mixture should be drunk immediately because it tends to gel rather quickly. During a fast, psyllium can be taken three to five times daily. Some people like to take an herbal laxative the night before beginning a fast in order to initiate the elimination process.

Other useful detoxification products include proteolytic enzymes (pancreatin or bromelain), probiotics, vitamin C, and chlorophyll. Probiotic supplements, containing *Lactobacilli* and Bifidobacteria, help to re-establish microorganism balance in the intestinal tract. Enzymes supplements can be useful to help break down and "digest" dead tissue and debris.

The use of vitamin supplements during a fast is usually not advised, with the exception of vitamin C. Vitamin C is considered a useful detoxifier.

Spirulina, chlorella, alfalfa, Swedish flower pollen extract, and the cereal grasses wheatgrass and barley grass may also be taken while fasting to provide concentrated nutrition without taxing digestion. The green food concentrates are also good sources of chlorophyll.

Vigorous exercise is not recommended during a fast, but stretching, yoga, deep breathing, walking, and fresh air can be very helpful. Sauna baths and dry brush skin massage may help to release toxins through the pores.

Modified Juice Fast

Liquids (1 ½-2 quarts daily)

A variety of:

Diluted fruit juice

Lemon water

Distilled water

Vegetable juice

Herb teas

Detoxification Supplements

Psyllium seed powder or husks

Herbal laxative

Probiotics

Vitamin C

Chlorophyll

Swedish flower pollen extract

Green food concentrates (spirulina, chlorella, wheatgrass, barley grass)

Proteolytic enzymes (pancreatin, bromelain)

What to Expect

If we are in tune with the body's signals, we will instinctively know when the time is right to end the fast. It is important that the fast be broken gradually, eating only small quantities of whole fruit, soups, and salads, over one or two days to allow the system to adjust to solid food. It would be unfortunate to end a fast with a case of indigestion. The end of a fast is a good time to make a commitment to eat sensibly and follow a natural foods diet. Some of the benefits from fasting are better health, increased energy, mental clarity, creativity and spirituality, and improved complexion and overall appearance.

Hunger might be experienced during the first day or two of the fast. After this time, hunger generally subsides. Toxins will be released, and a person may feel nauseated or experience mild headache, bad breath, or skin eruptions. Also, it is not uncommon to see unusual material expelled from the bowel. All of these manifestations can be symptoms of a toxic condition and an indication of the need to cleanse internally.

Often, those who fast remark that they have a lot more time on their hands. We don't often realize how much time we spend during the week shopping for, preparing, and eating food. The money saved can be put toward purchasing your fasting supplies.

Daylong or two-day fasts are ordinarily safe for an individual with an informed plan. Fasts of a longer duration should only be undertaken by those who are experienced and knowledgeable on the subject and who have qualified supervision. Fasting is not advisable for women who are pregnant or nursing or for anyone in a weak or debilitated condition. People with chronic ailments such as heart disease or diabetes, or those taking medication, should consult a physician. Fasting can affect one's response to medication, making some drugs dangerously potent in their effect.

Vegetable Broth for Fasting

2 large potatoes (unpeeled), chopped
2 celery stalks, chopped
1 large carrot (unpeeled), chopped
1 beet, chopped
6 cups water

Combine all ingredients in a stainless steel, enameled, or earthenware utensil. Cover and bring to a boil, reduce heat, and cook slowly for half an hour. Strain; store in refrigerator. Warm the broth before drinking.

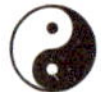 Yin-Yang Diet Recommendation

The body requires food and food abstinence. Restrict your food intake from early evening until breakfast. Consider a formal fast weekly, monthly, or when the seasons change. When properly executed, a fast can be a decisive step toward taking control over your health.

Chapter 8

Acid and Alkaline

pH Balance

Body chemistry is influenced by food, mood, and metabolic and muscular activity. Bodily fluids respond to these factors by fluctuating between acid and alkaline states. Acid foods (fruits and vegetables) are oxidized into alkalies, and alkaline foods (meats and grains) are oxidized into acids. In other words, the acids in fruits and most vegetables are used as fuel by the body, leaving behind alkaline elements (potassium, for example). Meats and grains, on the other hand, stimulate hydrochloric acid secretion by the stomach for their digestion and to kill microbial organisms. To be healthy, the human body must have a balance between acid and alkaline.

The measure of acidity or alkalinity of a solution is called pH (potential of hydrogen). On the pH scale, seven is neutral. Higher numbers indicate increased alkalinity while lower numbers represent increasing acidity.

A diet that is not balanced can stress body chemistry by causing extreme acidity (acidosis) or alkalinity (alkalosis). Each extreme has symptoms and can cause illness. For example, blood is always maintained at approximately 7.4 (slightly alkaline). The slightest deviation will cause trouble and eventually death. The typical Western diet, which is high in meats and grains and low in vegetables and fruits, is highly acid-forming.

When the acid level in the body is raised by muscular exertion or oxidation of protein and starches, the acids are broken down and excreted through the kidneys, lungs, and skin and neutralized or buffered by minerals (sodium, potassium, calcium, and magnesium).

If the kidneys have a hard time excreting excess acid, more alkalizing minerals are drawn from bone reserves. Recent studies suggest that too many grains and baked goods may lead to bone loss by creating an acid load. When tissues become overly acidic, calcium is pulled from the bones to neutralize it.

Potassium is essential for healthy blood pressure but also helps maintain our acid-base balance. Potassium citrate in particular appears to boost bone density by neutralizing excess acid in the body.

Swiss researchers gave 169 subjects either a placebo or enough potassium citrate to supplement their diets with 2,400 milligrams of potassium a day. After two years, the potassium takers had higher spine, hip, arm, and leg bone density than the placebo takers.[1] When US researchers gave men and women either a placebo or potassium citrate, those taking the potassium lost less calcium.[2]

The best approach to help maintain a normal pH is a low-stress diet properly balanced in Yin and Yang. (There are Yin and Yang in the acid-forming foods as well as in the alkaline-forming foods.) A low-stress diet is one that puts the least amount of strain on digestion and metabolism. It is not too extreme in Yin or Yang or any one type of food. In terms of volume, one part acid-forming to four parts alkaline-forming is best for physically active people who create more acid and need to alkalize themselves. For less active individuals, a one-to-two ratio is appropriate or even one-to-one at times.

Acid-Forming Foods

Meat

Dairy

Fish

Eggs

Grains, pasta, flour (except quinoa, buckwheat)

Peanuts

Nuts (except hazelnut, macadamia)

Seeds

Lentils

Pale beer

Cocoa

Alkaline-Forming Foods

Most fruits, fruit juices

Vegetables

Beans

Tofu (prepared with calcium sulfate)

Red, white wine

Mineral water

Note: Lists of acid/alkaline-forming foods often differ. The classifications presented here are based on a scientific formula calculated by Dr. Thomas Remer.[3]

Acid-Forming Elements

Phosphorous

Sulfur

Chlorine

Alkaline-Forming Elements

Calcium

Sodium

Potassium

Magnesium

The pH of urine gives an accurate index of the natural acid/alkaline cycles of the body. Checking urine pH tells us if we need to increase acid-forming or alkaline-forming foods. Urine pH generally fluctuates between 5.0 and 7.5. The ideal urine pH is believed to be in the range of 6.2 to 6.8 (mildly acid). This range is said to promote healing and building in the body while allowing for excretion of wastes.

In one study, smokers who had acidic urine smoked more than smokers with alkaline urine.[4] The study showed that they excreted more nicotine in acid urine. On the other hand, they smoked fewer cigarettes if they were made alkaline by taking baking soda (sodium bicarbonate). Since one of the main reasons smokers smoke is for the stimulus-barrier effect of nicotine, the study participants smoked less when they were alkaline and their blood and brain nicotine levels were higher.

Charting Your Urine pH

Charting your urine pH is an adventure in body communication. Keep a role of pH paper test strips with you and in your bathroom. Pass the test strip through the urine stream, shaking off any excess. When the color changes, match it with a color on the dispenser. Record the numbers on a sheet of paper or graph. Test your urine at your first urination in the morning to get a baseline. You can then test two hours after each meal to observe the effect your meal had on your pH. Initially, pH should be checked at each urination for several days to become familiar with patterns in your acid/alkaline cycles. It takes a while to determine if you lean toward acid or alkaline. After a while you will know if you are acid or alkaline just by your body's signals.

Urine pH fluctuates with meals and tends to be more acid in the morning and more alkaline in the evening. It is not unusual to go into an alkaline cycle within an hour after eating. Radical departures from these normal cycles indicate stressful body chemistry. Remaining at 5.0 to 5.5 throughout the day, for example, indicates acidosis whereas remaining at 8.0 or above is indicative of alkalosis. It is desirable to correct either extreme to minimize stress to the adrenal glands, which work with the kidneys to regulate acid-alkaline balance.

Symptoms of Acidosis

Frequent sighing

Increased heartbeat

Restlessness

Cold sweat

Dry skin, mouth

Hard stools

Diminished urination, perspiration

Sticky, sour taste in mouth

Halitosis (bad breath)

Adrenal fatigue

Antidotes—Reduced animal protein and grain consumption; increased alkaline-forming foods (vegetables, steamed spinach, grated radish, miso soup and moderate amounts of fruit); apple juice (½ cup at a time); ½ teaspoon bicarbonate of soda in water at one-to-two hour intervals until urine pH registers alkaline;* cool temperatures, a cool shower, and deep breathing favor alkalinity.

* Unless you have acid indigestion (heartburn), avoid taking bicarbonate of soda (baking soda) within an hour or so of eating, since stomach acidity is needed for proper digestion.

Symptoms of Alkalosis

Muscle soreness, cramps

Stiff creaking joints

Bursitis

Bone spurs

Edema (especially swollen hands)

Allergies

Menstrual problems

Hyperventilation

Restlessness, excitability

Numbness, prickly sensations

Increased respiration

Circulatory problems

Discomfort after eating (due to lack of stomach acid)

Lowered resistance (bacteria, viruses, fungi, parasites, and other microorganisms tend to thrive in an alkaline environment)

Antidotes—Increased acid-forming foods; unsweetened cranberry juice (½ cup at a time); raw apple cider vinegar (1 teaspoon to 3 tablespoons in water before or after meals); moderate exercise will also reduce alkalinity.

Note: Prolonged alkalosis can cause a drop into acidosis due to adrenal cortex exhaustion.

Life on Earth depends on appropriate pH levels in and around living organisms and cells. With increasing industrialization over the past one hundred years, the pH of our oceans has dropped from 8.2 to 8.1 because of increasing CO_2 deposition. This has a negative impact on life in the oceans and may eventually lead to the collapse of the coral reefs.Also, the pH of soils in which plants grow can have considerable influence on the mineral content of food.[5]

☯ Yin-Yang Diet Recommendation

Become familiar with your acid-alkaline states by periodically checking your urine pH. Heed the signs of the body, and make the necessary dietary adjustments to keep yourself balanced.

Chapter 9

Basic Meal Balancing

Feel Full and Satisfied

The *Yin-Yang Diet* is about achieving nutritional balance by combining foods of various flavors, colors, energies, and actions. It consists basically of selecting at least one Yin food and at least one Yang food for each meal. There is no one percentage or quantity of Yin-Yang foods to eat. Instead, the focus is on eating foods that support your Yin-Yang needs.

The *Yin-Yang Diet* is a plant-based diet, one in which plants provide more weight, volume and calories than animal foods. (It's not a vegetarian diet, though vegetarian principles can be applied.) It's a diet that will satisfy your appetite while helping you maintain a healthy weight. One reason diets don't work is that they severely limit the amount and types of food one can eat. Studies show that eating wholesome natural foods, like whole grains (high in fiber), vegetables and fruits (high in fiber and/or water content) don't need to be severely restricted because they fill you up but don't contain a lot of calories. Studies also show that it is not the number of calories one eats that makes a person feel satisfied but rather the weight and volume of food.[1]

Another benefit of eating a plant-based diet is that plant fibers foster growth of beneficial gut microbes. Recent research suggests that substances secreted by probiotic bacteria may cause less fat to accumulate, boost calorie burning, and increase satiety.

One striking difference between Asian-style diets and a Western diet is the meat portion. In American restaurants, twelve-ounce steaks are the norm, whereas traditional Asian meals typically contain 2-3 ounces of meat. Eating a 12-ounce steak will send a person into extreme Yang and craving chocolate cake from the dessert menu. The *Yin-Yang Diet* recommends small portions of meat. A meal properly balanced in Yin and Yang will leave you feeling balanced, full, and satisfied.

Eggs can also be easily consumed in excess especially when the diet already contains other animal protein. The Chinese consider one egg sufficient for several people (as it is mixed into eggdrop soup or fried rice).

A prerequisite of the *Yin-Yang Diet* is that you prepare most of your meals. In our modern world where two-thirds of us are either overweight or obese, we are tempted to just go to a fast-food drive-through, heat up a frozen dinner, or eat out at restaurant. In healthy populations, people grow their food and prepare their own meals. Though we don't all have gardens, it's a basic Yin-Yang principle that you must expend energy to earn your meal. Eating must be balanced with physical activity. Otherwise, unhealthy, excess body fat will accumulate.

Combine Yin Foods with Yang Foods

Modern nutrition science is based on knowing the chemical composition of foods, whereas Asian nutrition is based on food energetics and the forces of Yin and Yang. Combine Yin foods with Yang foods at most of your meals. Throughout the meal, different dishes will be more Yin or more Yang than each other. What matters is the overall balance. In the *Yin-Yang Diet*, there are no good foods or bad foods. However, extreme Yin or Yang foods should only be eaten in moderation, especially if one suffers from an illness. The majority of one's food intake should consist of non-extreme foods, which have more subtle actions. Swinging from extreme to extreme can keep us balanced, but it is more gentle and healthier to maintain balance by moving between less extreme positions.

All foods can be classified on a scale according to their varying degrees of Yin or Yang. The double end arrow indicates Yin on one end and Yang on the other end. On the furthest extreme of Yin are fruit, sugar, and alcohol. Eggs, meat, and salt are on the furthest extreme of Yang. Yin foods tend to be moist and watery, low in calories and rich in potassium, while Yang foods tend to be dense and dry and high in calories and sodium.

Yin←Alcohol Sugar Honey Butter Oil Fruit Nuts Tofu Vegetables Seeds Beans Milk Yogurt Cheese (Soft) Sea Vegetables Neutral (Balance Point) Whole Grains Fish Poultry Cheese (Hard) Eggs Red Meat Coffee Salt→Yang

You should strive for Yin and Yang balance at each meal. But if you only have Yin foods at one meal, your next meal should favor Yang foods.

Examples of Yin and Yang Pairings (Combine at least two elements)

- Fish + beans
- Beans + rice
- Oatmeal + cranberries
- Chicken + vegetables
- Tofu + rice

After a meal, assess how you feel. About one to three hours after eating, you'll know if you had the right Yin-Yang ratio. The right combination will leave you feeling balanced and satisfied. After a while, you will develop a heightened sense of awareness of how the Yin-Yang ratio affects you physically and mentally.

Right Yin-Yang Ratio

Appetite—feel full and satisfied, no sweet craving, not hungry again soon after eating

Energy—restored energy and sense of well-being

Mental—emotional uplift, mental clarity

Wrong Yin-Yang Ratio

Appetite—physically full but still hungry, desire for sweets, hungry again soon

Energy—fatigue, sleepiness, hyper but exhausted underneath

Mental—mentally slow, poor focus, depressed or anxious, irritable

Include Five Flavors

Have you ever noticed how we tend to crave salty snacks after eating sweets? This is the body's attempt to maintain balance, and an example of Yin-Yang interplay. Ideally, a meal should provide all five tastes to reflect the Yin-Yang dynamic and provide different beneficial actions. The five flavors are sweet, sour, salty, bitter, and pungent. (Schizandra, a tonic herb, is said to contain all five flavors.) Throughout a meal, the five tastes may each predominate within one or more dishes, but overall the meal should balance out. The tastes that predominate in Western diets are sweet, salty, and sour. By consuming an excess of these tastes, we are eating an imbalanced diet.

Sweet—Sweet is both calming and energizing. The following foods are considered sweet: apple, apricot, cherry, date, fig, and many other fruits that also have a sour flavor, beet, carrot, cucumber, eggplant, potato, squash, sweet potato, grains (rye, quinoa, and amaranth are also bitter), honey, molasses, rice syrup, all legumes (beans, peas, lentils), meat, fish, and dairy.

Sour— Sour helps with digestion of fats and protein and assimilation of minerals, and it lowers the glycemic (blood sugar) response of carbohydrates. The following foods are considered sour: citrus fruits, other sour fruits, yogurt (sour and sweet), sourdough bread (sour and sweet), and apple cider vinegar (also bitter).

Salty—Salty stimulates digestion. The following foods are considered salty: Celtic salt, seaweed, soy sauce, and celery (also bitter).

Bitter— Bitter increases appetite and promotes digestion, and bitter herbs are sometimes used to relieve constipation. The following foods are considered bitter: dandelion, arugula, endive, alfalfa, romaine lettuce, white pepper, bitter melon, and dark chocolate; green tea and the grains rye, quinoa, and amaranth are both bitter and sweet.

Pungent— Pungent stimulates digestion and circulation. The following foods are considered warming pungents: ginger, cinnamon, clove, black pepper, hot peppers, cayenne, horseradish, nutmeg, cardamom, garlic, and onion. Examples of cooling pungents include: peppermint, white pepper, and radish. Note: cayenne and other peppers are extremely warming and can change to a cooling effect after thirty minutes or so (Yang shifting into Yin).

Include Five Colors

The five colors should also be present: red, yellow, green, white, and tan/dark.

Red (nourishes the heart)—The deep red, blue, and purple colors of fruits and vegetables come from water-soluble pigments with powerful antioxidant properties that complement the fat-soluble carotenoids. Red foods include tomato, beet, red bell pepper, and berries. Berries contain high levels of anthocyanidins. Red tomatoes contain high levels of the carotenoids beta-carotene and lycopene.

Green (nourishes the liver)—Chlorophyll, a fat-soluble pigment, is found in green vegetables such as broccoli, parsley, and leafy greens. Chlorophyll, the "blood" of plants, stimulates hemoglobin and red blood cell production. Research indicates that chlorophyll can latch onto carcinogens (cancer-causing agents) in the digestive tract and prevent their absorption. Broccoli, cabbage, kale, and Brussels sprouts (cruciferous vegetables) contain highly researched sulfur compounds that participate in liver detoxification and help to prevent cancer, especially breast cancer.

Yellow (nourishes spleen and stomach)—There are many yellow-orange foods to choose from, including yellow and orange squash, carrots, corn, sweet potatoes, yams, citrus, tropical fruits, and egg (yolks). They are good sources of carotenoids, including beta-carotene, which the body converts into vitamin A. Egg yolks contain the carotenoid lutein.

White (nourishes lungs)—cauliflower (a cruciferous vegetable), daikon, white beans, tofu, jicama, turnip, soymilk, fish, dairy, and the protein-oil shake.

Tan/dark (nourishes kidneys)—grains, whole-grain bread, black beans, black sesame, mushrooms, seaweed. They contain antioxidant trace minerals and cholesterol-lowering fiber and phytosterols.

Another Yin-Yang aspect of food is whether it is wet or dry. By balancing dry foods against wet foods, you can correct any excessive dryness of the body or excessive dampness of the body. Perfect color, flavor, and texture are the highest compliments one can pay to a chef!

Seasonal Eating

The summer season and hot climates tend to bring out heat signs in everyone, regardless of constitution. Increasing cooling foods, such as salads and fruits, and decreasing warming foods, such as meats and animal fats, is beneficial to everyone at this time. Raw vegetables and fruits, steamed vegetables, and fish are appealing in summer. Summertime foods include lettuce, tomato, melon, cucumber, summer squash, and bell peppers. Be especially careful not to overeat on hot summer nights.

In the more Yin winter, we require more warming or Yang foods, especially on cold winter mornings. Winter foods include oatmeal, soups, stews, cooked vegetables, beef, chicken, and eggs. Both salty and bitter foods are appropriate for winter. However, use salt with discretion because too much causes water retention and coldness. Follow the example of nature, and eat seasonally available foods as they come and go throughout the year.

Eating Out

Diners and fast-food restaurants are representative of everything that is wrong with the modern Western diet. However, some places offer healthful fare, and you do have choices from the menu. Eating out should be an exception and not the rule. If eating out is a rare occasion, it's OK to relax your standards. No one is going to criticize you for having a piece of cake on your birthday. It's not what you do on occasion that counts. It's what you do as a routine.

Raw or Cooked?

Raw food diets are increasing in popularity, as witnessed by the emergence of raw food "cook" books and restaurants. In general, this can be considered a healthful trend, but as with many diets, they are often taken to extremes.

A raw food diet basically consists of salads, fresh juices, and sprouted seeds, grains and legumes. For some, it might include raw eggs, unpasteurized dairy products, fish (sushi, for example), and rare steaks.

On the plus side, uncooked foods contain enzymes, the life force in growing plants, which pre-digest food when thoroughly chewed. When foods are heated above 105 °F, they begin to lose enzyme activity. By 118 °F, most enzymes are completely destroyed. When you put a cooked potato in the ground, it rots. When you put a raw potato in the ground, it grows into a new plant. Enzymes can also be obtained by eating cultured foods, such as yogurt, miso, and kimchi, as bacteria contained in them produce enzymes. Raw foods also provide nutrients that may otherwise be lost in cooking water or destroyed by heat. Health food pioneers, like Bernard Jensen, have recommended a diet as much as 70 percent raw, while today some enthusiasts advocate raw foods exclusively.

To my knowledge, no human studies have been done on raw food diets. However, we can apply Yin and Yang principles here. A diet that is mostly raw is ideal for summer. It's cooling and good for inflammations and overweight bodies. On the other hand, raw foods may not be helpful for cold/damp conditions like fungal infections (Candida, for example). Also, too much raw food can actually weaken digestion ("digestive fire") and may harbor parasites and harmful bacteria.

Cooking food can actually make some nutrients, beta carotene and lycopene for instance, more available to the body by breaking down fibrous plant cell walls. One study found that men who consumed more lycopene from cooked tomato products like spaghetti sauce experienced a reduced risk of prostate cancer compared to those who seldom ate the foods.[2] The effect, however, was not observed in those consuming raw tomatoes.

Cooking can also inactivate undesirable compounds in certain raw foods. For example, goitrogens, found in cruciferous vegetables such as broccoli, cabbage, and cauliflower, can inhibit thyroid function. If these are eaten in large quantities, as one might be inclined to do on a vegan diet, they might cause weight gain by slowing metabolism.

For best health, we need to strike Yin and Yang balance by eating a diet that contains both raw and cooked food. Diets that are exclusively raw might be beneficial and therapeutic in the short-term for weight loss and for ailments caused by dietary overindulgence, but in the long run, exclusively raw diets can be harmful to the body.

How to Get More Vegetables in Your Diet

A recent survey found that 42 percent of Americans eat fewer than two servings of vegetables and fruits a day. Moreover, the vegetable serving was often French fries. Another survey found that 45 percent of Americans fail to eat *any* fruits or veggies on a randomly selected day. Studies suggest we may need as many as 7-10 servings per day, mainly for their fiber and antioxidant content, to reduce the risk of cancer and other diseases. This may sound like a lot, but a serving is one cup of leafy greens, a half-cup of cooked vegetable, or one small whole fruit. The latest government guidelines no longer stress numbers of servings but now emphasize that half of one's plate consists of vegetables and fruits.

There are some vegetables and fruits that have been strongly associated with disease prevention. They are spinach (vision), cruciferous vegetables (broccoli, cauliflower, cabbage, Brussels sprouts) (cancer), tomatoes (cooked, sauce) (prostate cancer), pomegranate (blood pressure, artery plaque), blueberries (brain) and prunes (dried plums) (osteoporosis).

Make sure you shop twice a week so you'll have plenty of fresh produce in your refrigerator, though frozen is acceptable, too. Try a new vegetable every so often. Think vegetables every meal. A large salad is perfect for a hot summer day, and soups and stews are ideal for cold weather. I've included tasty vegetable recipes in Appendix 3.

☯ Yin-Yang Diet Recommendations

Prepare as many of your meals as you can at home.

Include both Yin and Yang foods at most meals.

Include five flavors at meals.

Include five colors at meals.

Chapter 10

Meal Balancing for Your Constitution and Condition

Balance for Who You Are

In addition to being aware of the Yin-Yang nature of foods, remember that you the eater bring a Yin or Yang element to the table. Therefore, all foods should be evaluated with regard to the particular balance of the person eating it. As you develop greater sensitivity to the qualities of each food you eat, you will then begin to intuitively select those that create a healthy balance for you. Simply becoming aware of an imbalance is the first step toward becoming balanced. Ultimately, whether a food is beneficial or not is determined by its effect on your body.

Every individual differs in their age, sex, constitution, and present condition. Smaller personal adjustments should be made in diet to suit these differences. People engaged in different activities have different dietary requirements, too. More physical and social activities such as gardening, farming, sports, public speaking, or business management are more Yang, and they require a slightly more Yang diet to sustain this activity. This can be achieved with more chicken and fish in the diet. More mental, emotional, intellectual, and philosophical work such as art, writing, administration, religious and spiritual activities, and social work are more Yin, and those require a slightly more Yin diet to promote these abilities. This can be achieved with little or no animal foods.

Balance for Your Present Condition (Shifting Yin Toward Yang, or Yang Toward Yin)

When we become imbalanced in Yin and Yang, we suffer an excess of one and a deficit of the other. Since we rarely see purely Yin or Yang conditions but rather a combination of both, we should consider our main symptom first and our constitution second.

Symptoms of Excessive Yin/Deficient Yang

- Chill
- Dislike of cold/attracted to warmth
- Weak, frail
- Withdrawn
- Soft voice
- Shallow breathing
- Depression
- Bodily excretions: clear urine, watery stools, thin/watery mucus, dampness
- Sexually under-aroused

Remedies

1. Use warming foods, longer cooking, fewer raw foods
2. Use hot peppers (in moderation) and warming spices: ginger, clove, cinnamon
3. Drink less fluids
4. Eat oats, quinoa, sesame, walnut, brown rice, cabbage, kale, mustard greens, parsley, garlic, onions, unrefined sweeteners (in moderation), butter, and moderate amounts of animal protein

Symptoms of Excessive Yang/Deficient Yin

Dislike heat/attracted to cool

Dryness

Aggression

Loud voice

Heavy breathing

Anxiety

Bodily excretions: dark urine, constipation, thick/yellow mucus

Sexually over-aroused

Remedies

1. Use more relatively cooling foods: raw, sprouted, salads, steaming and simmering are OK
2. Avoid meat, animal fat, alcohol, coffee, spices
3. Emphasize liquids
4. Eat grains and legumes—wheat, millet, mung beans, tofu

On cold winter days or when experiencing symptoms of cold, favor more cooked foods, soups, stews, and warming herbs and spices. On hot summer days or when experiencing symptoms of heat, favor more raw and cool foods, like fresh fruit, raw vegetable sticks and pieces, and large salads.

A Healthy Weight

It's no secret. Obesity is epidemic in the US. Two-thirds of us are either overweight or obese. It's not just a cosmetic issue. Being overweight increases the risk of heart disease, diabetes, and some types of cancer, and it shortens life.

The weight-loss equation sounds simple: Burn more calories than you take in. But in spite of the longstanding eat-less-move-more prescription, obesity rates continue to climb. This has caused researchers to look at not just how many calories people eat and burn, but also what kind of food the calories are coming from and how the body processes them.

Nutritionists used to think that a calorie is a calorie. In other words, it didn't matter if it was coming from cheesecake or carrots. If you ate too many calories, you would accumulate body fat. Turns out, this idea is too simplistic.

A propensity for obesity and the diseases that accompany it is largely due to the quality of carbs and the hormones that regulate their metabolism. For example, if you are eating the majority of your carbs as flour products, pastries, sodas, fruit juices, and sugary breakfast cereals you are stressing your blood sugar control mechanisms. Refined carbs are devoid of fiber. Thus, they tend to spike the blood sugar level, causing the pancreas to secrete excessive amounts of the hormone insulin. Insulin facilitates the entry of blood sugar (glucose) into muscle cells to be burned for energy but also to be stored as fat. Furthermore, the constant bombardment of glucose and insulin creates an imbalance in the pleasure centers of the brain that can lead to food addiction, which is not unlike tobacco, alcohol, or cocaine addiction.

In contrast, if you eat carbs in their natural state, such as from whole grains, brown rice, oats, vegetables, and whole fruits, their fiber content allows them to enter the bloodstream at a slower rate. This gradual rise in blood glucose prevents the surge of insulin and excessive fat storage.

Whether the carbs are cooked or raw also affects fat metabolism. Raw foods take more energy to digest than cooked foods. So, if you are overweight you should be eating more salads than a person with a normal body weight.

An important benefit of eating a plant-based diet is that plant fibers foster growth of beneficial gut microbes. Recent research suggests that substances secreted by probiotic bacteria may cause less fat to accumulate, boost calorie burning, and increase satiety. Calorie counts do not consider any of these factors.

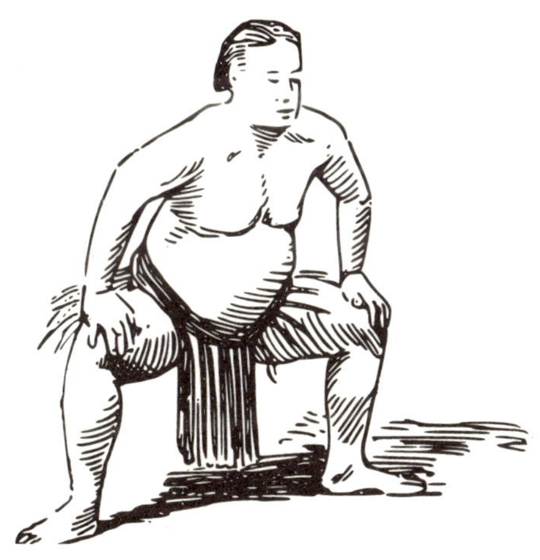

Do You Eat Like A Sumo Wrestler?

The weight-loss equation sounds simple: burn more calories than you take in. But it's not just about decreasing food intake and becoming more active. It's also about ***how*** we eat and ***what*** we eat. This is evident in the dietary habits of Japanese sumo wrestlers whose goal is to gain as much weight as possible, usually about four hundred pounds.

Sumo wrestlers skip breakfast then work-out on an empty stomach. By working out on an empty stomach, they secrete more cortisol, a stress hormone that ramps up appetite. Also, they eat just one or two large meals a day, mostly higher carb with some meat and little to no fat. Consuming most of one's calories in one or two meals results in more fat storage compared to dividing calories among three or four smaller meals. With the majority of calories coming from starchy carbs like bread, potatoes, rice, and noodles, body fat is more easily increased. Carbs are the body's preferred fuel for energy. But if we don't burn them in physical activity, they are stored as body fat. It may seem counterintuitive to limit fats in the sumo diet, but some fats promote loss of body fat by increasing heat (thermogenesis) and calorie burning. In simple terms, the body is reluctant to give up its stored fat when deprived of essential fatty acids found in seeds, nuts, olives, avocado, and fish. The small amount of meat in the sumo wrestler's diet provides protein needed to build muscle. However, body fat is more important to them because it occupies more space and is less metabolically active than muscle. Lastly, sumo wrestlers eat a TON of calories and drink beer with their meals, then go right to sleep for three to four hours during the day or overnight after the last meal. (No explanation required.)

So, if you want to reduce body fat, do the opposite of what sumo wrestlers do. On the other hand, if you want to literally throw your weight around, the sumo diet is for you!

Balance for Your Constitution

A person with a Yin constitution can have a higher proportion of Yang foods in their diet than a person with a Yang constitution. Conversely, a person with a Yang constitution should favor more Yin foods.

Do You Have a Yin or Yang Constitution?

Your constitution determines your overall Yin-Yang dietary balance. Everyone has both Yin and Yang aspects, though each of us can be broadly categorized as either Yin- or Yang-dominant. We need both Yin and Yang foods at most meals. However, for nutritional balance, a person with a Yang constitution will require a greater proportion of Yin foods, just as a Yin person will require a greater proportion of Yang foods.

Yin-Yang Self-Analysis

Yang

Large bones, sturdy frame

Aggressive, gregarious

Ruddy complexion

Easily angered, fiery disposition

Propensity for physical activity

Testosterone dominant

Sexually aggressive

Illnesses tend to be acute

Yin

Thin bones, frail frame

Passive nature

Pale complexion

Not easily angered, tendency toward fear, anxiety or melancholy

Low testosterone or estrogen dominance

Gentle, soft-spoken

Patient, nurturing

Sexually passive

Illnesses tend to be chronic

☯ Yin-Yang Diet Recommendation

Fine-tune your Yin-Yang food intake according to your activity, present condition, and constitution.

Chapter 11

Yin Tonics and Yang Tonics

Adaptability

Throughout the world, indigenous people have developed an intimate relationship with the plants around them. Thousands of years of experiential knowledge of herbs form the basis of many traditional healing systems. About 30 percent of pharmaceutical drugs are derived from plants. Unlike drugs, herbs are generally far less toxic to the system and can be taken long-term because they are balanced by many ingredients.

Chinese herbalism is the most developed herbal system in the world. An important distinction from other herbal systems is that it emphasizes the promotion of health rather than the elimination of disease. Since the introduction of acupuncture to the West, more Westerners have been turning to Chinese herbs because of the vast scope of experience in China. In every province, there are large schools of traditional Chinese medicine, research institutes, and teaching hospitals where thousands of practitioners gain training in the use of herbs.

In the West, we generally think of herbs as being medicinal or culinary. Chinese medicine categorizes herbs into three categories: Kingly (non-toxic), Ministerial (moderately toxic), and Servant (toxic). This roughly corresponds to foods, over-the-counter drugs, and prescription drugs. Kingly herbs are used routinely to reinforce the body's resistance. Ministerial and Servant herbs are used temporarily as treatment for emergencies and threatening symptoms or to offer immediate comfort for a patient. Like drugs, they cannot create health. The body must expend precious energy trying to rid itself of a drug. Drugs help manage and prevent life-threatening symptoms, but if they were good for us, we'd take them all the time.

Tonic Herbs

Tonic herbs are Kingly herbs that benefit well-being much more than common herbs. They may be thought of as superfoods that nourish and protect us. Tonics are restorative substances that strengthen and invigorate organs or the entire body. A tonic is something that improves well-being. In traditional Chinese medicine, to tonify means to augment, replenish, and strengthen. Chinese tonic herbs balance Yin and Yang, gradually bringing the body into a natural state of balance. Herbal researcher Daniel Mowrey associates the following ten properties with tonics:[1]

1. Return and maintain balance (homeostasis) to the body.
2. Greatly increase metabolic production of energy (through mitochondria, for example).
3. Raise resistance to infectious disease.
4. Decrease anxiety and stress, and increase ability to function, as well as to rest and sleep.
5. Provide antioxidant effects.
6. Increase the body's ability to form new muscle tissue and to lose weight by burning more calories.
7. Regulate digestive processes.
8. Provide components that strengthen the heart and normalize blood circulation.
9. Help maintain the health of the liver and related organs and glands.
10. Help keep bowel movements regular and smooth.

Tonic herbs are broadly considered adaptogens, substances that help the body adapt to physical, mental, and emotional stress by restoring altered body conditions back to normal. Rather than addressing specific symptoms, adaptogens bolster our natural ability to deal with all types of stress and rebalance whatever is out of whack. The term adaptogen was not coined until the 1960s by Drs. Israel Brekhman and Nikolai Lazarev, two Russian scientists who were studying plants. They found that certain herbs were particularly good at adapting to and surviving in harsh conditions and had been helping humans to do the same for a long time. The Soviet Union was performing studies from the 1950s until the 1980s on the effects of herbs on athletes and cosmonauts to establish the adaptogenic classification. They said that to be classified as an adaptogen the plant had to meet three characteristics. It had to be non-toxic to the body's physiology, it had to increase the body's resistance to adverse influences, and that the plant would have an overall normalizing effect without aggravating or having side effects or an adverse reaction.

A long and healthy life is very much dependent on our ability to adapt to stress. Adaptogens are bi-directional, which means if you are wound up it's going to bring you down to a normal level, but if you are down in the dumps it's going to bring you up. Adaptogens either reduce stress reactions in the alarm stage or prevent or retard the exhaustion stage.

Yin and Yang tonics are an integral part of the *Yin-Yang Diet*. Unlike medicinal herbs, which are taken temporarily when we are ill, tonic herbs can and should be taken routinely for health maintenance and superior health.

Yin tonics help with the accumulation of energy and moisture. They are analogous to the upswing of a pendulum, which gathers energy. Yin tonics are herbs and foods that are nourishing, moistening, cooling, or anti-inflammatory. They are the most important anti-aging, longevity herbs and foods. Everyone can benefit from a Yin tonic. Choose one or more Yin tonics, depending on your need. You may also supplement with a combination formula.

Yang tonics help us utilize energy. They are analogous to the downswing of the pendulum, releasing the energy. Yang herbs are activating, drying, warm, or hot. They are the sexual, athletic tonics. Yang tonics stimulate metabolism, build muscle, reduce body fat, and strengthen bone, the lower back, and joints. Choose one or more Yang tonics. You may also supplement with a combination formula. Note: *Yang tonics should be used in moderate quantities by those with a Yang (hot) constitution or symptoms of excess Yang, such as fever. For those who are extremely Yin-deficient, it is best to build Yin before adding Yang tonics as they might exacerbate their condition.*

Descriptions of the tonic herbs appear in Appendix 5. When you learn about their amazing properties, it might be hard to choose, though some might stand out for your particular needs. I suggest you experiment by trying different tonic herbs. Eventually, you'll find what works best and feels right for you. Each tonic has unique properties, which can make it easier to pick one. Tonic herbs are very safe, but as with anything, it is wise to begin with a lower dosage to establish that they agree with you. Periodic evaluations and reconsiderations are also advised.

Herbal Preparations

Herbs are consumed fresh or dried and as fluid or solid extracts. When we make a cup of tea, we are creating an extract called an *infusion*. We discard the solid, fibrous waste in the tea bag and consume the active ingredients dissolved in the hot water. Alcohol or other solvents can also be used to extract plant constituents. If the solvent is evaporated off, the result is a dry extract that can be encapsulated or pressed into tablets.

Herbal extracts come in various concentrations. For example, a 4:1 extract indicates it takes four pounds of crude, powdered herb to make one pound extract. The term "standardized" refers to an extract guaranteed to have consistent levels of active compounds so that it can be dosed more accurately. This is important in clinical studies requiring herbal preparations that do not vary. Just as vitamin levels vary from one apple to another, herbal constituents can vary from batch to batch. A standardized ginkgo biloba extract is often expressed as a 50:1 concentration containing 24 percent ginkgoflavonglycosides (active ingredients). Milk thistle extract might be expressed as a 30:1 concentration containing 80 percent total flavonoids.

As an herb goes through multiple extractions to standardize specific active ingredients, other constituents in the herb are removed or reduced. For this reason, some traditional herbalists prefer non-standardized products containing all of the plant's constituents.

☯ Yin-Yang Diet Recommendation

Supplement your diet with one or more Yin or Yang tonic herbs.

Note: If you have a medical condition or are pregnant, lactating, trying to conceive, under the age of 18, or taking medications, consult your healthcare professional before using herbs.

Chapter 12

Twenty Principles of the Yin-Yang Diet

Staying in Balance

Include both Yin and Yang foods at most meals.

Throughout the meal, different dishes will be more Yin or more Yang than each other. What matters is the overall balance.

Prepare most of your meals at home.

It's a basic Yin-Yang principle that you must expend energy and earn your meal. Eating must be balanced with physical activity. Otherwise, unhealthy, excess body fat can accumulate. Part of that physical activity should be spending an hour or so preparing your meals. More and more, we are cooking less and consuming food prepared by someone else outside of our own kitchens. In 2015, the US Commerce Department released data showing that, for the first time ever on record, consumers spent more money at restaurants and bars than at grocery stores.

Never go more than four or five hours without eating unless fasting.

Divide your daily food intake into three meals per day. If you go too long without eating, you are more likely to binge on unhealthful snacks or overeat at your next meal. If your meal is properly Yin-Yang balanced, you will experience peak levels of blood sugar, hormones, and neurotransmitters about two hours later, what elite athletes call being in "the zone."

Eat until 80% full.

With that in mind, you are not in danger of overeating and becoming uncomfortable and lethargic. (It takes energy to digest.) Eat just enough to get you to your next meal—not so much that you are not hungry at the next mealtime, and not so little that you get hungry before mealtime. Your system more likely can handle whatever you eat and remain balanced if you don't stuff yourself.

Practice mindful eating, eat slowly, relax, chew food well, and enjoy meals.

Mindful eating is a slower, more thoughtful way of eating. You are eating with the intention of caring for yourself and with the attention necessary to enjoy your food and its beneficial effects. When you eat slowly, you are less likely to overeat. It takes about fifteen minutes for your brain to get the message that you're full.

Have the protein-oil shake three to five days a week.

This is one of the most important principles of the *Yin-Yang Diet*. It helps to build healthy new tissue, maintain a steady blood sugar level, manage weight, and support liver detoxification.

Include both land and sea vegetables in your diet.

Sea vegetables, or sea greens, are far more concentrated in minerals than land vegetables. Sea vegetables include any number of highly nutritious marine plants like kelp, arame, dulse, hijiki, kombu, wakame, and nori. (See Appendix 3 for recipes.)

Balance meals with five flavors.

Ideally, a meal should provide all five tastes (sweet, sour, bitter, salty, pungent) to reflect the Yin-Yang dynamic and provide different beneficial actions. Throughout a meal, the five tastes may each predominate within one or more dishes, but overall the meal should balance out.

Incorporate herbs and spices into your diet.

We all know something about the health consequences of vitamin and mineral deficiencies. But is it possible to have a spice deficiency? Culinary herbs and spices are believed to be key factors in traditional diets of healthy populations and are lacking in the typical American diet. Herbs are the leaves of the plant, while spices come from the roots, bark and seeds. Curry is a famous Asian herb and spice blend that incorporates a dozen or more herbs, including turmeric. Studies on turmeric's cancer-fighting qualities have been published in major medical journals. Many of these studies were spurred by the observation that India, where spices like turmeric form an important part of the diet, has a rate of colon, breast, prostate, and lung cancer that is ten times lower than that of the US. Herbs and spices you should regularly include in your diet are ginger, cinnamon, clove, cilantro, green tea, rosemary, oregano, dill, basil, parsley, and mint.

Eat more warming foods in winter and more cooling foods in summer.

On cold winter days or when experiencing symptoms of cold, favor more cooked foods, soups, stews, and warming herbs and spices. On hot summer days or when experiencing symptoms of heat, favor more raw and cool foods, like fresh fruit, raw vegetable sticks and pieces, and large salads.

Limit refined carbohydrates and added sugars in your diet.

Refined carbs include white flour products, polished rice, cookies, pies, cakes, pastries, candy, sugary breakfast cereals, and soda pop. Sugar is the most Yin of all foods.

Avoid high-sodium processed foods.

Main sources of high-sodium are canned soups and vegetables, frozen entrees, salty snacks, and fast foods.

Avoid deep-fried foods, trans fats, and rancid fats.

Trans fats (partially hydrogenated oils) are often found in margarines and snack items. Rancid fats are present in old opened bottles of oils, ground meat, and leftovers. Brief stir-frying with small amounts of oil is acceptable.

Avoid smoked, salt- and nitrate-cured meats and fish including most hot dogs, bacon, sausage, salami, ham, and smoked salmon.

Sodium nitrite is a preservative used to stabilize the red color in cured meat. Without nitrite, hot dogs and bacon would look gray. Adding nitrite to food can lead to the formation of small amounts of potent cancer-causing chemicals called nitrosamines. Smoking of food with wood smoke may increase the risk of certain cancers.

Limit consumption of grilled or barbecued meats.

Chemicals produced during grilling or barbecuing of red meat, poultry, lamb, pork, and fish are carcinogenic (damaging to

DNA and contributors to cancer). Fat drippings from high-fat grilled meats combined with the heat from the flame or coals can produce potentially carcinogenic chemicals called PAHs (polycyclic aromatic hydrocarbons). PAHs can be released into the smoke and also form directly on the meat if it is charred. To minimize PAHs, avoid placing meat directly over the coals or heat source where smoke is heaviest. Lean meats, poultry, fish, vegetables, and veggie burgers are better choices to avoid PAHs. When meat is cooked to extremely high temperatures, the heat creates potentially carcinogenic HCAs (heterocyclic amines), and the levels of HCAs can increase the longer the meat is exposed to the high temperatures. Seafood and vegetables are less likely to form HCAs. A marinade helps prevent HCAs from forming during cooking.

Do not eat a large meal within three hours of bedtime.

If you are hungry at bedtime, have a small snack (about 200 calories) to prevent your blood sugar from falling during the night. A drop in the blood sugar level during the night can interrupt sleep by causing you to wake up.

Drink 8-12 ounces of water upon arising, between meals, and after exercise.

You may add a squeeze of lemon or an ounce of fruit juice for flavor. You may sip a beverage during meals to refresh the palette.

Supplement your diet with tonic herbs.

When we think of herbs, we often think of the culinary herbs that account for the distinctive flavors of various ethnic cuisines. Medicinal herbs might also come to mind, which are taken to fight colds, flu, and other illnesses. But unlike medicinal herbs, which are taken temporarily, tonic herbs can and should be used routinely for health maintenance and superior health.

Practice occasional fasting to correct dietary indiscretions.

The most natural way to fast is to stop eating early in the evening until you "break-fast" the following morning. However, fasts of a longer duration can be helpful at times.

Always choose organically grown foods when possible.

Billions of pounds of agricultural chemicals are sprayed on crops annually in an effort to increase productivity and improve the appearance of food. Ironically, pests of all kinds are destroying more crops each year as they become chemical-resistant. Pesticides may be intended for pests, but they also affect humans. Pesticide exposure is a risk factor for many health problems including neurological diseases and some forms of cancer.

Although the insecticide DDT was banned in 1975, virtually everyone carries it in their tissues today. Researchers have found that fatty breast tissue from women with malignant breast tumors contained more than twice as much DDT byproducts as breast fat from women of the same weight and age who did not have cancer.

The National Academy of Sciences reports that an average American consumes approximately 40 milligrams of pesticides per year in food alone and carries about 100 milligrams permanently in body fat. Children, whose bodies are still developing, are especially at risk from pesticides, as are pregnant women, whose unborn children are extremely susceptible to damage from these toxic chemicals.

Organic foods are those grown and brought to market without the use of chemical pesticides and fertilizers. However, because our environment has become so polluted, there is no way that organic foods can claim to be 100 percent pesticide-free.

Organic produce often has higher nutrient levels. In addition, organic farms are more hospitable to critical pollinators like bees and butterflies. Organic foods tend to cost a little more because more of the farming work is done by hand, such as weeding.

Each year, the Environmental Working Group, a not-for-profit environmental research organization, releases a list of fruits and vegetables that are most and least contaminated with pesticide residues. By avoiding some of the most contaminated produce and favoring the least contaminated, you can reduce your exposure to pesticides by almost 80 percent.

Appendix 1

Beverages

Juices

Fresh juicing provides a high concentration of active enzymes and essential vitamins and minerals along with the cooling properties of raw vegetables and fruits. Juicing can make it easier for us to meet recommended servings for vegetables and fruits. Juicing also concentrates the sugars in fruits and sweet vegetables like carrot and beet. For this reason, juices from these foods should be limited to a quarter cup at a time or combined with non-sweet vegetables such as celery and spinach. Juices lack fiber, which is discarded as pulp. So if you juice, make sure to get adequate fiber from other plant sources. Bottled fruit juices are high in sugar, so be sure to dilute them at least 50/50 with water if you drink them at all. Generally, it is better to eat the whole fruit, which is mostly water. Juicing is often recommended in conjunction with a fast and as a dietary therapy for cancer and other diseases.

Sodas

The occurrence and death rates of various degenerative diseases such as diabetes, obesity, cancer, heart disease, liver and kidney disease, and Alzheimer's disease continue to rise. This suggests something is terribly wrong with our diet and lifestyle. Consumption of sugar from sodas is believed to be a major contributor. I see families coming out of warehouse stores wheeling out case stacks of Coke and Pepsi. An all-too-familiar scene is a family sitting around the dinner table with a 2-liter bottle of soda. They don't drink water!

The problem is not so much the sugar itself but the unhealthy quantities people consume. A 12-ounce can of soda contains about 39 grams of sugar—almost ten teaspoons of sugar. Most of us would not think of eating ten teaspoons of sugar from the sugar bowl. Yet, that is what we consume in each can.

Fruits, vegetables, and whole grains naturally contain sugars. However, the sugar in whole foods is accompanied by all the nutrients (fiber, vitamins, minerals, etc.) necessary to metabolize the sugar properly. Fiber, for example, slows the absorption of sugar, preventing it from being dumped into your bloodstream all at once. Thus, we avoid stressing our blood sugar control mechanisms.

A good rule is don't try to satisfy your thirst with sweet beverages. Make sure you drink enough water for that purpose. Then, if you still want something sweet and bubbly, limit it to half a cup.

Green Tea

Green tea (*Camellia sinensis*) is a non-fermented tea in which the fresh young leaves are lightly steamed or pan-heated and then dried. It is one of the most popular beverages worldwide. Green tea's health benefits have been known for more than 4000 years, and they are said to exceed the benefits of other teas. Studies have shown convincing results for its many health properties, including cellular, cardiovascular, immune and nerve cell health.

The power of green tea comes from its high levels of polyphenol antioxidants. Green tea supplies significantly more health benefits than black tea due to its higher content of free polyphenols. Within 40 minutes of consumption, we get a boost in antioxidant power in our bloodstream and within 60 minutes, an upregulation of DNA repair.

Green tea is one of the most potent cancer inhibitors in your diet. In mice, it provides protection from all stages of cancer, including initiation, promotion, and progression. Studies show that green tea polyphenols inhibit cancer by blocking the formation of cancer-causing compounds such as nitrosamines, suppressing the activation of carcinogens and detoxifying or trapping cancer-causing agents.[1] Nitrosamines are found in processed meats (smoked, canned, and preserved), grilled meats, and tobacco smoke. Although important in fighting all types of cancers, green tea is especially important in preventing breast and prostate cancers.[2,3] Green tea consumption may be one of the major reasons for the low rate of cancer in Japan.

Although green tea contains caffeine, even sensitive individuals usually find that drinking it does not produce the excessive stimulation that the same amount of caffeine from coffee can induce. This is probably due to the fact that green tea also contains the amino acid theanine, which is known to facilitate relaxation. Studies show that theanine induces alpha brain waves, a mental state that is also experienced while meditating or being hypnotized. The relaxed state of alertness created by green tea makes it a good choice for creative thought processes rather than coffee, which speeds the ability to perform mental tasks.

Green tea is the perfect beverage to consume with meals because it helps to protect against toxins while it increases calorie expenditure. In European trials, subjects taking green tea extract burned more fat calories compared to those taking a placebo.[4]

Got Matcha?

Matcha is a powder specially made from young green tea leaves. Matcha is twenty times more potent than regular green tea due to the way it's processed. The plants are kept in shade for two to four weeks before harvesting, which boosts the chlorophyll and antioxidant levels. The leaves are then steamed, dried, and ground with a stone grinder. The labor-intensive process makes matcha more expensive than regular green tea. You might think of it as the "champagne" of green tea.

Matcha is the preferred product in Japanese tea ceremonies. It's said that the Samurai would drink it before battle for hours of sustained energy. Because you are consuming the whole tea plant rather than a tea infusion, the caffeine is more slowly released into your system. A teaspoon (2 grams) of powder contains about 70 milligrams of caffeine.

Matcha powder can be added to recipes or a protein shake. You can make a matcha latte with hot milk and swap it out for your morning coffee. For a cold beverage, shake or blend it with ice and a sweetener. Since matcha is stimulating and cleansing, I suggest starting with a half teaspoon.

Yerba Mate

Yerba mate (*Ilex paraguareinsis*), a member or the holly family, is a tea-like beverage made from the leaves and stems of a rainforest tree, native to the subtropical rainforests of Paraguay, Brazil, and Argentina. It boasts abundant quantities of vitamins, minerals, amino acids, and antioxidants. Yerba mate may be comparable to green tea in its total polyphenol antioxidant content. Yerba mate is also known for its adaptogenic qualities, which include reducing the effects of stress. South American traditional herbal medicine employs yerba mate as a tonic, diuretic, stimulant, and aid to gastric functions.[5] It is also used to promote internal cleansing and the elimination of wastes from the body. In Germany and France, yerba mate is used as a weight-loss aid. Yerba mate, with naturally occurring caffeine, delivers both energy and nutrition.

Coffee and Caffeinated Drinks

While watching a Ken Burns documentary on the Civil War, I learned that the favorite beverage of soldiers, both North and South, was coffee—4 pints (2 quarts) a day. They would crush the beans with their rifle butts, and they often had to stretch it by adding ground peanuts or chicory.

Today, coffee is America's favorite beverage for energy and alertness, though it affects people in different ways. For people prone to insomnia or with conditions aggravated by stress, it is best avoided or enjoyed only in moderation.

Research out of Duke University found that people who consume caffeine may experience an increase in blood pressure, feel more stressed, and produce more stress hormones than on days when they abstain.[6] They concluded that any condition influenced by stress could also be aggravated by caffeine. In fact, the combination of caffeine, stress, and a tendency to hypertension can cause dangerously high blood pressure.

The effects of caffeine appear to persist until we go to bed, even if we don't consume any after one p.m. Caffeine has a half-life of four hours average. This means that however much caffeine you consume, it will take your body four hours to rid itself of half that amount. And four hours later, your body will contain only one-quarter of the original amount. Consequently, twelve hours after consuming caffeine, your body still contains one-eighth of what you first drank.

Coffee accounts for close to 75 percent of the caffeine we consume. There is some evidence that people who consume coffee or caffeine regularly have a lower risk of Parkinson's disease and gallstones compared to non-users. However, there is also a downside that is often ignored. Too much coffee or caffeine can cause panic attacks, anxiety, insomnia, diarrhea, heartburn, palpitations, increased blood cholesterol level, ringing in the ears, and disruption of circadian rhythm. Coffee has been specifically linked to fibrocystic breast, migraine, osteoporosis, infertility, pancreatic cancer, miscarriage, and, in men, weight-gain. The more coffee consumed, the greater the risk.

Some people rely on coffee to stimulate their bowels. It purges the bowels, which are often sluggish from a diet heavy in rich, processed, and greasy foods.

No one can tell you how much coffee is safe for you, so it's important to know your tolerance and use discretion. Some of us are fast metabolizers of caffeine while others are slow metabolizers, depending on the activity of a liver enzyme that detoxifies caffeine. Most health practitioners will tell you that one or two cups of coffee a day is reasonable, but for some (me included) that's too much. Coffee drinkers often say, "I need that morning cup to function" or "I cannot speak until I've had my coffee." The drug-like effect that it provides these frequent drinkers is actually a reversal of their withdrawal symptoms and a sign of addiction.

Many people mistakenly believe that coffee and high-caffeine beverages like Red Bull and Rockstar provide energy to the body. Although they contribute calories, the buzz we feel comes from caffeine's effect on the adrenal glands, which pump out adrenaline and other stress hormones that elevate blood sugar and blood pressure. In effect, caffeine forces your glands to work harder, so you use up your reserve of energy faster than you normally would. And there's a price to pay. With excessive use, caffeine just makes you nervous and more tired due to exhausted adrenals. The savings account, so to speak, is empty. That's why people eventually require as much as six or eight cups of coffee to get the same level of stimulation they used to get from one or two cups.

In TCM, judicious use of a stimulant would be when *chi* (energy) gets stuck, so to speak. It's used to jump-start or unblock the flow of energy. However, stimulants are not recommended if one is deficient, because they would further exhaust one's adrenals and exacerbate an already debilitated condition. I don't know of any traditional diet that recommends drinking coffee if you have a disease.

Bottom line: Know your tolerance for coffee and caffeine-containing beverages. Extreme foods should only be consumed in moderation, especially if you are dealing with health issues. Kicking coffee may not be pleasant. But once you are off the bean, you'll find that your energy is more consistent and on a higher level rather than peaking and dipping. Tonic herbs will help to wean you off caffeine. Try ginseng, ashwagandha, *Cordyceps*, *Rhodiola*, and *Eleuthero*. You won't feel a jolt, but you'll acquire calm, consistent energy, greater stamina, and an improved sense of well-being.

Alcoholic Beverages

Alcoholic beverages can be cooling (like beer) or warming (like brandy). The average person makes about one ounce of alcohol every day by normal metabolism.

There is substantial evidence for the benefits of alcohol consumption in moderation. People who drink light to moderate amounts of alcohol have a 25-40 percent lower chance of developing heart disease[7]. Moderation is defined as no more than one drink for women and two for men a day. (One drink is defined as 12 ounces of beer, 5 ounces of wine, or 1.5 ounces 80-proof liquor.) Alcohol thins the blood, making it less likely to form a clot that could block an artery, causing a heart attack or stroke. However, binging on the weekend because you've abstained all week will not provide protection. Binging interferes with coordination, takes its toll on your liver, increases the risk of certain cancers, and puts you and others at risk when you go behind the wheel.

Louis Pasteur, the French chemist credited for pasteurization, proclaimed that wine is the most healthful and hygienic of all beverages. Wine is an integral component of one of the most healthful and scientifically documented diets in the world—the traditional Mediterranean diet. This diet, initially researched during the 1960s, was consumed by people living in parts of Greece, Italy, and Spain. It consisted of seasonally fresh vegetables and fruits, grains, fish, olive oil, red meat only once or twice per month and, of course, red wine. At that time, people in this region enjoyed long lives and had a heart disease rate that was 90 percent lower than that in the United States.

The comparatively low rate of heart disease in France despite a diet that includes butter and cheese has become known as the "French paradox." Some experts have suggested that red wine makes the difference. Red wine contains a chemical called resveratrol that has been shown in animal experiments to greatly increase lifespan.

People drink alcohol for different reasons. As they say, some drink to remember, some drink to forget. It is a social lubricant that lowers inhibitions and allows boisterous or playful activities. It also acts as a stimulus barrier to filter out unwanted stimulation from the environment. The potential health benefits of alcohol can make it very appealing. But as we know, there is a dark side. Not everyone is able to practice moderation. For various physiological and psychological reasons, alcohol can be a deadly, addictive drug. It has caused much grief and ended the careers and lives of many good people.

How Much Water Do You Need?

We've all heard the 8 x 8 prescription—drink at least eight eight-ounce glasses (64 ounces) of water a day. But where did this rule originate, and what is the scientific basis? Several years ago, a kidney specialist looked into this matter. Turns out, a government report from 1945 stated that the body needs approximately 1 milliliter of water for each calorie consumed—about 8 cups for the typical 2,000 calorie diet. The report also included a key bit of information that seems to have been forgotten—that most of this quantity is contained in prepared foods. In other words, much of the body's water requirement will be obtained by consuming soups, juices, cooked grains, etc.

It's apparent that one's diet is a significant factor in determining how much water a person needs to drink in order to cleanse and stay hydrated. For example, those consuming high-protein diets need more water to dilute acid byproducts. The body's requirement will vary widely based on other factors, too, such as climate, condition, and activity level. Summer activities and sports can increase the risk of dehydration, particularly among children. Dehydration, if not treated, can lead to heat-related illness, such as heat cramps, heat exhaustion, and heatstroke.

Of course, too much of anything, including water, can be bad. I'm reminded of a radio contest several years ago in which a woman died of water toxicity by competing to see who could drink the most water. While some people brag about how much water they drink, others are putting their health at risk by not drinking enough. Elderly folks, for example, sometimes forget to drink, which can impair circulation by causing the blood to become too thick. While quantity will vary among individuals, three important times to drink water are upon awakening (to help elimination), between meals, and during and after physical activity. You may sip moderate quantities of beverages with meals to aid digestion and to cleanse the palette. However, too much liquid with meals is not good because it dilutes digestive secretions.

Appendix 2

Sweeteners

Sugars are identified by their suffix–*ose*. With few exceptions (like agave and corn syrup), most sweeteners and the naturally occurring sugars in fruit break down into roughly half fructose and half glucose in the body.

Sometimes we like to add a little sweetness to tea or a recipe. All sweeteners are best used in minimal amounts. Artificial sweeteners, such as acesulfame, aspartame, and sucralose, are not recommended because they might pose a slight cancer risk. More high-quality studies are needed.

Sucrose (Table Sugar)

Sucrose is broken down in the body to half fructose and half glucose. Highly refined sugars, like sucrose and fructose, contain none of the nutrients that normally accompany them in whole natural foods, which are necessary for the sugars to be metabolized properly. The American Heart Association recommends limiting refined sugar to six teaspoons (24 grams) per day for women and nine teaspoons (36 grams) for men.

Fructose

Fructose is a sugar that is slightly sweeter than table sugar (sucrose). When table sugar is digested, it breaks down into equal parts of fructose and glucose. Fructose occurs naturally in fruits and vegetables. Another major source is high-fructose corn syrup (HFCS). Fructose was once touted by some as a healthier sugar because it has a low glycemic index value (a measure of how quickly a food elevates blood sugar). However, large amounts from diets with a lot of added fructose, sucrose, and HFCS, are known to increase triglycerides and LDL cholesterol and may thereby increase the risk of heart disease. Large amounts may also increase abdominal fat and liver fat, which may increase the risk of diabetes and heart disease.

Honey

Honey is a food substance produced by bees. It is nearly all sugar (glucose and fructose). Honey contains some essential nutrients, including vitamin B2, B6, iron, and manganese. Raw honey is honey that has not been heated or filtered.

Honey has been used medicinally for millennia. Perhaps the best-known form of medicinal honey is Manuka honey. While all honey possesses some antibacterial properties, Manuka honey may be the most effective and most researched. Researchers note its effectiveness for wound treatments. In addition to its ability to destroy bacteria, a test-tube study found it highly effective against influenza viruses.[1] Other studies illustrate the use of Manuka honey for healing stomach ulcers and treating oral infections, and they also describe its anticancer benefits.[2] A rating system, called the unique Manuka factor scale (UMF) measures its therapeutic value. Manuka honey needs a minimum rating of 10 UMF to be considered therapeutic. Honey at or above that level is marketed as "UMF Manuka honey" or "active Manuka honey."

Raw honey is honey as it exists in the beehive without adding heat. Raw honey contains some pollen and may contain small particles of wax.

Infants can develop botulism after consuming honey contaminated with *Clostridium botulinum* endospores. While the risk honey poses to infant health is small, taking the risk is not recommended until after one year of age, and then giving honey is considered safe.

Maple Syrup

Maple syrup is derived from the sap of maple trees. Maple syrup is praised for its unique flavor. The most prominent sugar in maple syrup is sucrose. Maple syrup is generally low in overall micronutrient content, although manganese and riboflavin (vitamin B2) are at high levels, along with moderate amounts of zinc and calcium.

Maple syrup used to be labeled as Grade A or Grade B. Grade B is darker in color, is stronger in taste, and contains a higher amount of antioxidants. The stronger flavor is often preferred in recipes, whereas the lighter variety is used for pancake topping.

In 2014, for the sake of uniformity, Canada and the United States changed their laws regarding grading of maple syrup. Previously, each state or province had its own laws regarding color and taste. The new laws state that as long as the syrup does not have an off-flavor, is a uniform color, and is free of sediment, it can be labeled as one of four types of A grade: Golden Color with Delicate Flavor, Amber Color with Rich Flavor, Dark Color with Robust Flavor, and Very Dark with Strong Flavor If it doesn't meet these characteristics, the syrup is classified as processing grade or substandard.

Grade A

1. Golden Color and Delicate Taste
2. Amber Color and Rich Taste
3. Dark Color and Robust Taste
4. Very Dark Color and Strong Taste

Labeling laws prohibit imitation syrups from having "maple" in their names unless the finished product contains 10 percent or more of natural maple syrup. "Pancake syrup," "waffle syrup," and "table syrup" are substitutes, which are less expensive than maple syrup. In these syrups, the primary ingredient is usually HFCS, and they are usually thickened. Imitation syrups are generally cheaper than maple syrup, with less natural flavor. In the United States, consumers generally prefer imitation syrups, presumably because of the significantly lower cost and sweeter flavor.

Agave

Agave (pronounced *uh-GAH-vay*) syrup (or nectar) is a natural sweetener with a pleasant neutral taste. Agave is native to the hot and arid regions of Mexico and the Southwestern United States. Agaves are large, spiky plants that resemble cactus or yuccas but are actually succulents similar to *aloe vera*.

Agave syrup is 1.4 to 1.6 times sweeter than sugar and may be substituted for sugar or honey in recipes, though it is slightly thinner. Its color varies from light- to dark-amber, depending on the degree of processing. Agave has a higher fructose content (up to 60 percent) than any other common sweetener, more even than HFCS.

Rice Syrup

Rice syrup is a natural sweetener made from cooked rice that is treated with enzymes to turn the starches in the rice into sugars. It can be used like honey, molasses, and other liquid sweeteners. Rice syrup can be used as a cup-for-cup replacement for other liquid sugars. Compared to other sweeteners, the taste of rice syrup is mildly sweet. Rice syrup is essentially all glucose in that the sugars in rice syrup are broken down in the body to pure glucose. Rice syrup is popular in macrobiotic diets.

Molasses

Molasses is a by-product of cane sugar refining. It was popular in the Americas prior to the 20th century, when it used to be a common sweetener.

To make molasses, sugar cane juice is extracted and boiled to concentrate it. The third boiling of the sugar syrup yields a dark, viscous, strong-tasting liquid called blackstrap molasses. Blackstrap molasses is very nutritious and has long been sold as a dietary supplement. Unlike highly refined sugars, blackstrap molasses contains significant amounts of vitamin B6 and minerals, including calcium, magnesium, iron, and manganese. One tablespoon provides up to 20 percent of the Recommended Daily Value of each of those nutrients. Blackstrap molasses is also a good source of potassium. Blackstrap molasses is significantly more bitter than regular molasses.

Sucanat

Sucanat stands for sugar cane natural. It is dehydrated sugar cane juice, which retains the molasses. It is one of the least-refined sugars. Sucanat contains trace amounts of iron, calcium, vitamin B6, potassium, and chromium. It has a deep brown color and a distinct natural molasses flavor. Sucanat replaces brown or white sugar on a cup-for-cup basis. It works well in chocolate-based recipes, baked goods, BBQ sauces, and marinades.

Turbinado Sugar

Turbinado, or raw sugar, is a type of brown sugar that retains some of the molasses of cane sugar. It contains minor nutritional value and mineral content. Brown sugars that have been only mildly centrifuged or unrefined (non-centrifuged) retain a much higher degree of molasses.

Coconut Sugar

Coconut sugar is another alternative to cane sugar. It is a rich unrefined brown sugar with a deep caramel flavor. Coconut sugar is produced from the juice of cocnut flower blossoms, and its nutritional profile is richer than other sweeteners. Coconut sugar is 70–79 percent sucrose and only 3–9 percent each of fructose and glucose. Coconut sugar has a glycemic index value of 35 compared to 55 for honey and 68 for cane sugar, which means it is less apt to spike the blood sugar level. It works well in baked goods and on oatmeal, and it is also commonly used to sweeten Asian dishes, sauces, and beverages. It replaces brown or white sugar on a cup-for-cup basis.

Natural Sugar Substitutes

Stevia

Stevia is a non-caloric herbal sweetener derived from *Stevia rebaudiana*. In Japan, stevia has been widely used as a sweetener (including by Coke®) for many decades. The sweet-tasting compounds are glycosides, which have up to 150 times the sweetness of sugar. Stevia's taste has a slower onset and longer duration than that of sugar, and it has a slight bitter aftertaste. I find that it works well as a sweetener for iced tea. At typical sweetening quantities, stevia appears to be very safe. Studies are conflicting, but some suggest that stevia may lower postprandial (after meal) blood glucose levels by 18 percent.[3]

Xylitol

Xylitol is one of a number of natural sugar substitutes called sugar alcohols found in many fruits and vegetables. Sugar alcohols, such as xylitol, sorbitol, and erythritol, are commonly used in sugar-free products. Xylitol has roughly the same sweetness as sugar with 40 percent fewer calories and no aftertaste. It may be substituted for sugar on a 1:1 ratio. Xylitol does not crystalize as much as sugar, so it will not work well in peanut brittle or hard-candy recipes.

Unlike sugar, xylitol does not cause or contribute to tooth decay. Xylitol has negligible effects on blood sugar and insulin. The only downside is that it can cause intestinal discomfort and diarrhea if more than 25 grams are consumed in a day. Do not give xylitol to dogs because it is toxic to them.

Monk Fruit Extract (Lo Han Kuo)

Monk fruit is the fruit of *Momordica grosvenori*, a plant that grows in mountainous regions of Southern China. Monk fruit contains mogrosides, which are responsible for its characteristically intense sweet taste. An enzymatic and water extraction process results in sweetness that is 200300 times sweeter than sugar. The mogrosides, however, are not recognized by the body as sugars. They are non-caloric and have little effect on blood sugar or insulin levels.

Appendix 3

Recipes

Many of the recipes are simple and easy to prepare. Others a bit more complicated. Some of the recipes do not specify number of servings or quantities of ingredients as I leave the proportions up to you. All of the recipes have been tested and have received rave reviews from friends and family. I hope you enjoy them as well.

VEGETABLES

Kale and Black Olive Puree

Inspired by an award-winning Japanese chef.

Kale
Canned black olives, drained
Melted butter
Garlic salt

Bring a pot of water to a boil. Cook kale for about 5 minutes or until tender. Drain. Puree all ingredients in food processor.

Steamed Spinach with Garlic

Spinach
Garlic clove
Olive oil
Salt to taste

Peel and finely chop one garlic clove. Sauté garlic in a little olive oil for 1 minute. Rinse spinach. Add wet leaves to pan. Cover and steam for about 2 minutes.

Smashed Potatoes

2 medium potatoes
2 tablespoons butter
1 tablespoon Half and Half
1 tablespoon chopped parsley
1 teaspoon creamed horseradish
1 garlic clove, pressed
Salt and pepper to taste

Cut unpeeled potatoes into quarters. Bring pot of water to boil and cook potatoes for 10-15 minutes or until tender. Drain potatoes. Mash the potatoes in the pot with a masher. Add rest of ingredients. Mix well.

Roasted Pee Wee Potatoes with Rosemary

No need to cut these bite-size potatoes.

Small, whole potatoes
Sprinkling of extra virgin olive oil
Fresh or dried rosemary
Salt and fresh-ground pepper

In a mixing bowl, mix ingredients to coat. (Rub the rosemary between your finger tips to release its essence.) Transfer to a pan and bake at 425 degrees F. for 25 minutes or until soft.

Broccoli with Pickled Onion

Unadorned cooked broccoli is fine. But sometimes you want a different flavor.

Bite-size broccoli florets
Red onion, thinly sliced
¼ cup vinegar

Boil or steam broccoli for 5-7 minutes al dente. Separate onion rings. In a small saucepan, bring vinegar to a boil. Add onion rings. Simmer onion for about 2 minutes or until soft. Drain. Sprinkle onions on top of broccoli.

Stuffed Zucchini Boats

2 zucchini squash
½ c. finely chopped onion
Olive oil
2 tablespoons cottage cheese
1 egg, beaten
1 cup bread crumbs*
2 tablespoons grated parmesan cheese
1 tablespoon chopped parsley
Paprika
Salt and pepper to taste

Slice zucchini boats in half lengthwise. Place in a pan of boiling water and simmer 5-7 minutes or until pulp in center is soft. Remove zucchini from pan and allow to cool. Scoop out pulp with a teaspoon to make hollow boats. Reserve pulp. Heat a little olive oil in a pan. Sauté onion for 1 minute to soften. Stir in zucchini pulp, egg, cottage cheese, parmesan cheese, parsley, salt and pepper. Stir in enough bread crumbs to thicken the mixture until tacky and not wet. Fill zucchinis with stuffing, heaping in center. Dust zucchinis with paprika and place under pre-heated broiler for 2-3 minutes until slightly browned and crusty.

*You can make your own bread crumbs instead of buying packaged. Toast a few slices of bread. Allow to cool. Coarsely chop in a blender.

Steamed Vegetable Platter

2 cups chopped vegetables:
Broccoli
Carrot
Onion
Red potato
Cabbage or bok choy

Place all vegetables in a steaming basket, except cabbage/bok choy. Bring an inch of water to a boil in a soup pot. Place basket in the pot. Cover, reduce heat and simmer for 8 minutes or until crisp/ tender. Add cabbage or bok choy. Simmer for another 2 minutes. You may serve with a peanut or plum sauce for dipping.

Broccoli and Water Chestnuts

A simple vegetable side with complimentary textures and flavors.

Broccoli, cut into bite-size pieces
1 eight-ounce can of water chestnuts

Cook bite-size pieces of broccoli in boiling water for about 5 minutes or until crisp/tender. Add water chestnuts for one minute to heat. Drain.

Green Beans with Ginger

Goes good with Poached Fish.

Fresh green beans, ends trimmed
Fresh ginger root, peeled and cut into matchstick pieces (about 1 teaspoon per serving)
Toasted sesame oil

Drop beans into a pot of boiling water for about 5 minutes or until tender. Heat a little sesame oil in a skillet. Sauté ginger for 1 or 2 minutes. Turn off heat and add drained beans to skillet. Mix to coat.

Sautéed Shiitake Mushrooms

Shiitake is Japan's number one agricultural export and the most cultivated, popular and researched exotic mushroom. It is famous for its immune-enhancing properties. Sautéing shiitake mushrooms is uncomplicated. It only requires a hot pan and some oil to make the most of their smoky, rich flavor.

8 ounces fresh shiitake mushrooms
2 tablespoons olive oil
2 cloves garlic, chopped
Salt
Lemon juice

Cut off the mushroom stems and slice them diagonally. Slice the mushroom caps about ¼-inch thick. Heat the oil in a skillet. Add the garlic and cook and stir for about 1 minute, taking care that it doesn't burn. Add the mushroom caps and stems and cook over medium-high heat for about 3 minutes, until they are soft. Add a little more oil if they become too dry. Season with salt and a squeeze of lemon juice to taste.

Serves 4

SALADS

Red Potato and Green Bean Salad

Great for a summer picnic or pot-luck

1 ½ lbs. red potatoes, quartered
¾ lbs. green beans
1 small red onion, chopped
½ cup packed, fresh basil leaves, chopped

Dressing:

2 tablespoons vinegar
2 tablespoons mustard
2 tablespoons lemon juice
1 garlic clove, peeled and minced
Dash of Worcestershire sauce (optional)
1/3 cup olive oil
Salt and pepper to taste

Trim ends from green beans and cut in half. Boil or steam potatoes for 15-20 minutes or until soft but not mushy. (Insert a fork to test.) Add beans to pot for last 8-10 minutes. Cook until crisp/tender. Cool under tap or in ice water. Combine potatoes, green beans, onion and basil in a large bowl. Mix in dressing. Serve cool or room temperature.

Serves 6

Carrot Salad

This simple salad offers a fresh, unique flavor without oil or salt.

4 large carrots, shredded/grated
3 scallions (green onions), sliced
3 tablespoons chopped parsley
Juice of 1 lemon
1 teaspoon grated orange rind
2 tablespoons water
¼ teaspoon cayenne
½ teaspoon cumin powder
Vinegar to taste

Serves 4-6

Romaine Salad

This simple salad combines sweet, sour and bitter flavors. Dress with olive oil and balsamic vinegar.

Romaine lettuce
Red bell pepper
Jicama sticks
Grated carrot

Tomato and Cucumber Platter

1 tomato, sliced
1 Persian cucumber, sliced
Top with 1 teaspoon capers

Deluxe Kale Salad

Kale is a nutrient-dense cruciferous vegetable providing vision-supporting carotenoids and liver-detoxifying sulfur compounds. Vegetables, fruits, seeds, nuts—this delicious salad will leave you feeling very satisfied and extremely well-nourished!

1 bunch kale, finely chopped
2 medium carrots, grated
2 oranges, peeled and cut
3 scallions, sliced
3 tablespoons dried cranberries
3 tablespoons candied walnuts or pecans
Sprinkle of toasted sesame oil
Sprinkle of lemon juice
Sprinkle of sesame seeds or Eden Shake®
Sesame and Sea Vegetable Seasoning
Salt to taste

Serves 6

Spinach Salad

This delightful salad combines vegetable root, stalk and leaf. Combine ingredients in your desired proportions. Dress with a little olive oil and balsamic vinegar.

Spinach
Apple
Celery
Radish

Shiitake, Enoki, and Tofu Spring Rolls

Enjoy the fresh flavors of mint and cilantro in these spring rolls, which make great finger food for dipping. Serve them for a casual lunch or dinner, or as an appetizer.

Spring Rolls:

1.75 ounces enoki mushrooms
6 fresh large shiitake mushrooms, sliced
½ teaspoon olive oil
2 ounces thin rice noodles
8 large rice paper wrappers
6 ounces prepared fried tofu, cut into 8 thin slices
4 leaves romaine lettuce, cut in half lengthwise, then sliced widthwise into thin strips
Chopped fresh cilantro
Chopped fresh mint

Dipping Sauce:

3 tablespoons soy sauce
2 tablespoons water
1 tablespoon sugar
2 teaspoons lemon juice
½ teaspoon chili paste

To make the spring rolls, cut off and discard the tough bottoms (about 1 inch) of the enoki mushrooms. Separate the bunches, then separate the mushrooms. Cut the mushrooms into thirds. Fill a small saucepan with water and bring to a boil over high heat. Add the shiitake mushrooms and simmer for 1 minute. Remove the mushrooms with a slotted spoon and set aside. Add the enoki mushrooms to the boiling water and simmer for 1 minute. Drain and set aside. Fill a medium saucepan with water. Add the oil and bring to a boil over high heat. Add the noodles, decrease the heat to medium-high, and cook for 7 to 10 minutes, or until tender but firm. Drain in a colander. Rinse with cool water and drain again. Let the noodles air-dry.

Pour warm water into a large, shallow bowl until it is half full. Soften each rice paper wrapper, one at a time, just until pliable, by briefly immersing it in the warm water. (Do not allow the wrapper to absorb too much water or it will be difficult to work with.) Transfer the wrapper to a plate. Arrange some of the mushrooms, tofu, noodles, lettuce, cilantro, and mint in a row on the lower third of the wrapper. Carefully fold the bottom edge of the wrapper over the filling. Fold in the sides and continue rolling up from the bottom. Repeat the process with each of the remaining wrappers.

To make the dipping sauce, combine the soy sauce, water, sugar, lemon juice, and chili paste in a small bowl and mix well. Divide the sauce equally among 4 small serving dishes.

Just before serving, slice each spring roll in half crosswise. Serve with the dipping sauce.

Tip: Prepared fried tofu and rice paper wrappers are available in Asian markets, well-stocked supermarkets, and specialty stores.

Serves 4

Caprese Salad

Fresh buffalo mozzarella cheese balls (pearl size)

Tomatoes, sliced
Fresh basil leaves
Salt, pepper to taste

Place fresh basil leaves on tomato slices. Top with a mozzarella ball.

Deluxe Fruit Salad

Any combination of:

Apple, chopped
Seedless grapes
Strawberries, sliced
Tamarind orange segments

Seaweed "Caviar" Appetizer

Hijike is a rather expensive sea green, but nothing like real caviar (seasoned fish eggs), which can sell for tens of thousands of dollars for a kilogram.

¼ cup hijike
Water for soaking
1 tablespoon toasted sesame oil
1 shallot, minced (or 2 tablespoons minced onion)
1 garlic clove, minced
2 tablespoons shoyu (soy sauce)
Squeeze of lemon juice
Salt to taste
Sour cream

Soak hijike in water for fifteen minutes. Drain, squeezing out excess water. Finely chop hijike. Heat sesame oil in frying pan. Add hijike, shallot and garlic. Sauté for about 3 minutes. Add enough water to cover. Bring to a boil, add shoyu and simmer until liquid has evaporated. Transfer to a bowl and allow to cool slightly. Add lemon juice and salt to taste. Chill. Serve on crackers or toast triangles with sour cream.

Variation: Instead of lemon juice, try 1 tablespoon grated ginger root, squeezed to make juice.

Serves 6-8

Tofu Salad with Wakame

2 tablespoons wakame seaweed
1 lb. soft tofu, cubed
1 medium cucumber, diced
½ cup grated carrot
1 tablespoon sesame seeds
Salt to taste

Dressing:

2 tablespoons shoyu (soy sauce)
2 tablespoons water
Squeezed juiced from 2 tablespoons grated ginger root

Soak wakame for 10 minutes. Drain and chop into small pieces. Combine tofu, cucumber, carrot and wakame in mixing bowl. Pour dressing over salad and sprinkle with sesame seeds.

Asian Cabbage Salad

Cabbage, shredded
Carrot, julienned
Onion, sliced
Red bell pepper, sliced
Fresh cilantro, chopped
Fresh mint, chopped
Almonds or peanuts, chopped
Dressing:
Chili sauce
Lemon juice
Pinch of salt and sugar

SOUPS AND STEWS

Miso soup

4 cups water

1 strip wakame seaweed

1 medium onion, chopped

1 medium carrot, sliced

½ cup daikon radish, cut into matchsticks

1 tablespoon miso paste

1 cup fresh seasonal greens, chopped

1 ½ tablespoons tamari or soy sauce

Soak wakame in water for five minutes, then slice into small strips. Reserve soaking water for soup. Bring water to a boil. Add wakame, onion, carrot and daikon. Reduce heat, cover and simmer for 10 minutes. Add some of the hot liquid to a measuring cup. Stir in miso until dissolved. Add greens to soup. Cook 2 minutes more. Add miso and tamari.

Serves 4

Mexican Rice Soup

2 cups cooked brown rice
2 garlic cloves, peeled and minced
½ small onion, diced
1 small tomato, chopped
½ bell pepper, diced
½ cup tomato sauce
4 cups water or stock
1 teaspoon cumin
½ teaspoon oregano
3 tablespoons chopped fresh cilantro
Pinch of cayenne
Salt and pepper to taste

Place rice in soup pot along with water/stock, garlic, onion, tomato, bell pepper, tomato sauce, cumin, oregano, cayenne, salt and pepper. Bring to a boil. Simmer for 15 minutes. Garnish with cilantro.

Serves 4

Mediterranean Seafood Stew

A one-pot meal balanced in Yin and Yang

1 14-ounce can of minestrone soup
1 cup frozen seafood combination (shrimp, scallop, calamari)
Squeeze of lemon
Dash of Tabasco sauce
Dash of Worcestershire sauce
1 tablespoon fresh parsley, chopped

Place frozen seafood in a small saucepan. Add water and bring just to a boil. Drain. In a medium saucepan, combine all ingredients. Heat until hot.

Serves 1-2

Enoki and Asparagus Soup

Enoki mushrooms are long, thin white mushrooms that are often used in Asian cuisine. They have a crisp texture and are a good choice for grilling or adding to salads or soups. Enoki and asparagus combine well in this elegant soup. Be sure to add the enoki last so they retain a bit of their crunch. Nutritional yeast flakes provide a boost of nutrition and a chicken-like flavor.

3.5 ounce fresh enoki mushrooms
1 pound asparagus
6 cups water or vegetable broth
1 small onion, chopped
5 tablespoons soy sauce
1 tablespoon nutritional yeast flakes
1 teaspoon salt
Black pepper
3 tablespoons tapioca starch
3-4 tablespoons cold water

Cut off and discard the tough bottoms (about 1 inch) of the mushrooms. Separate the bunches, then separate the mushrooms. Break off and discard the tough bottom portion of the asparagus and peel the spears. Cut into 1½ inch-long pieces. Put the water in a large soup pot and bring to a boil over high heat. Add the asparagus, onion, soy sauce, yeast flakes, salt and pepper to taste. Decrease the heat to medium, cover and simmer for 15 minutes. Dissolve the tapioca starch in the cold water in a measuring cup or small bowl. Stir in the dissolved tapioca starch into the soup and cook for 2 minutes, stirring occasionally. Stir in the mushrooms and cook for 2 minutes longer.

Home Style Vegetable Soup

Use any fresh or frozen vegetables you may have on hand, such as:

1 medium onion, chopped

1 medium carrot, chopped

1 small potato, chopped

½ cup broccoli, chopped

1 small zucchini, chopped

1 small tomato, chopped or ½ cup canned

4 cups water

1 bay leaf

1 tablespoon chopped, fresh parsley

½ teaspoon dried Italian herb blend

Salt and pepper to taste

Bring water to a boil in a soup pot. Add all ingredients. Cover, reduce heat and cook 20 minutes. Remove bay leaf.

Serves 4-6

Japanese Ginger Stew

A hearty one-pot meal perfect on a winter day.

Large carrot, cut into matchsticks
2 cups packed spinach leaves
1 cup fresh cilantro, chopped
Red onion, sliced into half-rounds
4 ounces buckwheat soba
8 ounces seitan (wheat meat) or chicken breast, sliced
2 teaspoons fresh grated ginger
Sesame seeds
6 cups water
¼ cup tamari or soy sauce
Pepper to taste

In a soup pot, bring water to boil. Add carrot and onion. Reduce heat and simmer 10 minutes. Add spinach, cilantro, seitan or chicken, soba, ginger, tamari and pepper. Cook another 5-10 minutes. Top with sesame seeds.

Serves 4

CHICKEN

Baked Chicken with Chili-Garlic

1 skinless, boneless chicken breast

Chili-garlic sauce:

1 tablespoon olive oil

1 jalapeno pepper, seeded and chopped

1 garlic clove, peeled and chopped

1 teaspoon chili powder

Salt, pepper to taste

Pre-heat oven to 375 F. Rinse chicken breasts and pat dry with paper towel. Place chicken breast in shallow baking pan. In a small bowl or measuring cup, mix ingredients for sauce. Spoon sauce over chicken. Bake for 20-30 minutes. Do not overcook as chicken will be dry. When the flesh is no longer pink, and clear juice is released when pricked with a fork, it is done.

Serves 1

Korean Chicken and Vegetables

4 skinless, boneless chicken half-breasts, cut into 2-inch slices
1 medium onion, sliced
1 medium carrot, shredded
1 bell pepper, sliced
2 medium zucchini, shredded
2 scallions, sliced
2 tablespoon sesame seeds
2 tablespoons olive oil
3 tablespoons chicken broth or bouillon
1 tablespoon fresh grated ginger

Marinade:

3 tablespoons soy sauce
1 tablespoon toasted sesame oil
1 teaspoon honey
2 garlic cloves, finely chopped
Several grinds pepper

Cover chicken slices with marinade mixture. Let stand for 20 minutes. In a wok or large frying pan, cook chicken with marinade for about 2 minutes or until chicken turns opaque. Remove chicken from pan. Heat 2 tablespoons olive oil in pan. Add vegetables. Sauté for 3 minutes. Add chicken, sesame seeds and broth. Heat for additional 2 minutes.

Serves 4

FISH

Poached Fish with Vegetables

1 cup water

2 tablespoons tamari or soy sauce

4-6 ounces white fish (tilapia, sole, halibut or other) (frozen is ok, too)

1 cup thinly-sliced vegetables (fresh or frozen) such as zucchini, bell pepper and scallion

1 tablespoon peeled ginger root, cut into matchsticks

Fresh cilantro or parsley

Place fish in frying pan. Add vegetables and water and tamari. Bring to a boil. Cover and simmer gently for 5 to 10 minutes depending on thickness of fish. (Add an extra 2 minutes for frozen.) Move fish and vegetables to a platter. Spoon liquid over fish. Garnish with cilantro or parsley.

Variation: Instead of water and tamari or soy sauce, try white wine or chicken broth.

Serves 1

Sardine with Romaine Lettuce Appetizer

Sardine is a term denoting any small marine or freshwater fish, such as herring or menhaden. Ever wonder why they're packed so tightly in the can? It saves money. Turns out, the fish are less expensive than the oil used to fill up the can.

1 can small sardines (Tiny Tots® or King Oscar®)
Small hearts of romaine lettuce leaves
Grated parmesan cheese
Sriracha® sauce

Place one sardine on each small rib of romaine lettuce. Sprinkle with parmesan cheese and Sriracha® sauce. Watch them disappear.

Braised Salmon

Wild-caught salmon fillet
Butter or oil
¼ cup white wine or beer

Thaw salmon fillet if frozen. Pat dry with paper towels. Heat a small amount of butter or oil in a frying pan. Sauté salmon fillet briefly for 2-3 minutes skin-side up. Flip salmon fillet over, add wine or beer, and cover. Simmer for 3-4 minutes.

Serves 1

Curried Tuna Salad

6-ounce can of tuna, drained
1 hard-boiled egg, peeled and chopped
2 stalks of celery, chopped
¼ cup grated carrot
2 tablespoons currants
2 tablespoons mayonnaise
1 tablespoon chopped fresh parsley
1 teaspoon curry powder

Empty tuna into a mixing bowl. Break chunks into small pieces with a fork. Combine rest of ingredients, mixing well.

Serving suggestion: Place an ice-cream scoop serving on a bed of lettuce. Or cut a tomato into quarters but do not cut whole way through so it opens like a flower. Place a scoop of tuna into center of tomato.

Serves 2

Tuna and Pasta

1 cup spiral pasta
2.6 ounce packet of chunk light tuna
2 tablespoons extra virgin olive oil
2 scallions, chopped
Fresh cilantro, chopped
Salt
Pinch of cayenne pepper

Cook pasta in boiling water according to package instructions. Drain. Combine all ingredients.

Serves 1

Shrimp Scampi

1 ½ pounds jumbo, uncooked shrimp (20-40 shrimp) in shell
¼ butter
¼ cup white wine
1 garlic clove, crushed (optional)
Grated parmesan cheese
Paprika

Butterfly the shrimp: With small, pointed scissors, start cutting at the large end of the outside curve of the shell. Cut through the length of the shell down to the beginning of the tail. Then with a knife, cut through the length of the flesh just to, but not completely through, the underside. Rinse under tap, removing vein. Spread shrimp open and place in a large pot. Add butter, wine, and garlic. Bring to a boil over high heat. Cover and reduce heat. Cook until shrimp is opaque (about 5 minutes). Transfer to a platter and sprinkle with parmesan and paprika. Strain cooking liquid and pour into a small bowl for dipping.

Serves 4

Walnut-Crusted Salmon

Salmon and walnuts both deliver much needed omega-3 fatty acids.

Salmon fillets
Walnuts, finely chopped
Bread crumbs
Maple syrup
Olive oil
Lemon zest
Smoked paprika
Salt, pepper

Preheat oven to 375 degrees. Line a baking pan with foil. Place salmon in pan with skin side down. Mix walnuts, bread crumbs, maple syrup, oil, lemon zest, smoked paprika, salt and pepper. Distribute walnut mixture on top of each salmon fillet. Using your fingers, press gently. Bake for 10-15 minutes.

VEGETARIAN

Tofu with Miso-Seitan Sauce

1 lb. firm tofu cut into ½-inch slices

Sauce:

8 ounces seitan, finely chopped

½ cup minced onion

2 dried shiitake mushrooms, rehydrated and chopped

½ cup grated carrot

1 teaspoon fresh grated ginger

1 tablespoon miso, dissolved in ¼ cup hot water

1 tablespoon sesame butter (tahini)

2 teaspoons tamari

2-inch piece of kombu (seaweed)

4 cups water

Parsley for garnish

Place tofu in saucepan. Cover with water and bring to a boil. Turn off heat. (Tofu can also be grilled instead.) To make sauce, place onion, carrot, shiitake mushroom, seitan, kombu and water in saucepan. Add water. Bring to a boil and reduce heat. Simmer slowly until reduced to sauce consistency. Remove kombu. Stir in ginger, sesame butter, tamari and miso. Pour over tofu slices. Garnish with parsley.

Serves 4

Curried Rice

1 cup cooked brown rice
½ medium onion
½ medium apple
¼ cup cashew pieces
2 tablespoons dried currants or raisins
1 teaspoon curry powder
1 tablespoon ghee (clarified butter) or oil
Black pepper

Melt butter in a frying pan. Add onion, apple and cashews. Sauté for about 3 minutes or until softened. Add rice, currants or raisins, curry powder and pepper. Heat for 1-2 minutes. Serve with plain yogurt as a side.

Serves 1

Rice Au Gratin

2 cups cooked brown rice
2 stalks celery, finely chopped
½ medium onion, finely chopped
2 tablespoons dried shiitake or maitake mushroom (optional)
3 cups grated Swiss cheese
2 tablespoons chopped parsley
Olive oil cooking spray or olive oil
Paprika

Rehydrate mushrooms in a small bowl of water for about 10 minutes. Drain and chop. Heat a little olive oil in a frying pan. Sauté celery, onion, and mushrooms for about 3 minutes or until crisp/tender. In a mixing bowl, combine rice, celery, onion, mushrooms, grated cheese and parsley. Mix well. Grease two au gratin dishes with a little olive oil spray. Divide mixture into dishes. Dust with paprika. Place under a pre-heated oven broiler for 5 minutes or until cheese is melted.

Variation: Substitute pepper jack for Swiss cheese.

Serves 2

Vegetables Au Gratin

Broccoli, onion, carrot and potato, cut into bite size
Grated cheese
¼ cup almonds (try tamari almonds)
Olive oil cooking spray or olive oil

Drop vegetables into boiling water for 5 minutes or steam for 7 minutes. Lightly spray an oven dish with cooking oil spray or give a light coat with olive oil. Place alternate layers of vegetables, almonds and cheese in the dish. Place in a pre-heated oven broiler for 5 minutes to melt cheese.

Stir-Fried Rice with Ginger and Seitan

1 cup cooked brown rice
½ medium onion, chopped
1 stalk celery
1 teaspoon peeled and chopped ginger root
2 ounces seitan, chopped
1 tablespoon olive oil
Chopped parsley
Salt, pepper

Heat olive oil in wok or frying pan. Add onion, celery, and ginger root. Sauté for 3-4 minutes or until vegetables are softened. Stir in rice, seitan, and parsley. Cook for about 2 minutes or until heated.

Serves 1

Oatmeal with Chopped Nuts and Currants

Steel cut oats require a little more cooking time but they have a lower glycemic index than instant oats.

2 rounded tablespoons steel cut oats
1 cup water
Chopped almonds
Dried currants
1-2 tablespoon cream, Half and Half,
coconut creamer or plant milk

Bring water to boil in small saucepan. Stir in oats. Cook 10 minutes. Add currants for last two minutes of cooking. Top with nuts and cream.

Serves 1

Mock Meatloaf (Nut Loaf)

1 ½ cups walnuts, almonds or nut combination
2 cups chopped onion
¼ chopped parsley
¼ cup grated beet
1 cup diced tomatoes, drained (fresh or canned)
1 ½ - 2 cups whole grain bread crumbs
or crumbled shredded wheat
2 eggs, lightly beaten
1 teaspoon salt
Several grinds pepper
½ teaspoon Italian herb blend

Grind nuts in food processor or blender. Combine all ingredients except bread crumbs in a large mixing bowl. Add bread crumbs a half-cup at a time until mixture has consistency of ground meat. Pack mixture into a loaf pan and bake in pre-heated oven at 350 degrees for 50-60 minutes or until firm.

Serves 4

Brown Rice Burgers

2 cups cooked brown rice
1 cup finely chopped onion
2 garlic cloves, peeled and chopped
2 tablespoons sesame tahini
¼ grated carrot
2 tablespoons soy sauce
2 tablespoons chopped parsley
½ cup yellow cornmeal
¼ cup bread crumbs
1 egg, lightly beaten or egg substitute
1 tablespoon olive oil

Sauté onion, garlic, and carrot in olive oil for 3 minutes or until softened. Place cooked rice in a mixing bowl. Add cooked onion, garlic, and carrot. Add rest of ingredients. Mix well. Form mixture into patties using hands or a burger press. In a frying pan, sauté patties in a little olive oil over low heat for about 3 minutes each side.

Serves 6

Japanese Breakfast Bowl

½ cup (about ¼ ounce) dried shiitake mushrooms
¼ wakame
1 cup cooked quinoa or brown rice, warmed
½ medium carrot, julienned
2 scallions, sliced
1 tablespoon rice vinegar
½ teaspoon honey
1 tablespoon tamari
½ teaspoon fresh grated ginger
½ teaspoon toasted sesame oil
2 eggs, poached or fried
2 tablespoons sesame seeds

In a medium bowl, cover mushrooms and wakame with water and soak for 15 minutes. Drain and chop. In a mixing bowl, toss together quinoa or rice, carrot, scallions, mushrooms and wakame. In a small bowl, whisk together vinegar, honey, tamari, ginger and oil. Pour sauce over grain mixture. Divide mixture into two bowls. Top with egg and sesame seeds for garnish.

Serves 2

SMOOTHIE

Spinach-Cucumber-Apple Smoothie

Want to drink your salad? Unlike juicing, this blender smoothie retains all the fiber. Spicy, refreshing and delicious on a warm summer day. Provides three vegetable/fruit servings.

Blend:

1 apple, cored and chopped
½ cup chopped cucumber
1 handful spinach or other greens
2/3 cup ice cubes
½ cup cold water
1 teaspoon fresh, grated ginger
Squeeze of lemon
Pinch of cayenne

MENU SUGGESTIONS FOR YIN-YANG BALANCED MEALS

1. Tofu with Miso-Seitan Sauce
   Spinach Salad
2. Vegetables Au Gratin
   Mexican Rice Soup
3. Baked Chicken with Chili-Garlic
   Red Potato and Green Bean Salad
4. Curried Rice
   Plain Yogurt
5. Mediterranean Seafood Stew
   Deluxe Kale Salad
6. Poached Fish with Vegetables
   Green Beans with Ginger
   Brown Rice
7. Mock Meatloaf
   Broccoli with Water Chestnuts
   Romaine Salad
8. Korean Chicken and Vegetables
   Brown Rice
   Orange Segments
9. Tuna and Pasta
   Deluxe Fruit Salad
10. Walnut Crusted Salmon
    Mashed Edamame

Appendix 4

Food Facts, Fallacies and Controversies

Eggs

Easy to prepare and highly nutritious, eggs are one of America's most popular breakfast foods. They provide essential vitamins and minerals, unsaturated fats, lecithin, antioxidants, and protein. Their high-quality protein makes them the model for which other protein-containing foods are judged. Eggs also contain abundant amounts of the B vitamin choline, particularly important for brain function. Eggs can also be a good source of heart-healthy omega-3 fatty acids when the hens' diets are supplemented with flax or algae. The Chinese consider eggs a brain food.

In spite of their impressive nutrition profile, eggs have gotten a bad rap over the years. Because of their high cholesterol content, we were told to limit our consumption or avoid the yolk. The reasoning was that cholesterol is a component of the plaque that corrodes arteries, causing heart disease. But eating eggs is not likely to send your cholesterol levels soaring. Truth is, eggs do not contribute to heart disease. Most of the cholesterol in our bloodstream is homemade. In other words, our bodies make it.

When we eat cholesterol, the body makes less in a sort of feedback loop. Of greater concern is the saturated fat in our diets since this is the starting material for making cholesterol. Saturated fat is found primarily in fatty meats, butter, and whole milk products. Eggs are low in saturated fat.

Because eggs are rich in protein we don't need to eat a lot of them. They can be easily consumed in excess particularly if the diet already contains other animal protein. (Meat, eggs and dairy products contain arachidonic acid, a parent compound of inflammatory hormones.) The Chinese consider one egg sufficient for several people (as it is mixed into eggdrop soup or fried rice).

The healthiest ways to prepare eggs are soft-boiling and poaching. Boiling cooks them at a lower temperature than frying. This method prevents the cholesterol and fats from oxidizing and makes them more digestible. It is also less destructive to the antioxidants. Remember Rocky Balboa downing all those raw eggs as part of his training program? It's ok to have a raw egg in your shake, but there's a slight risk of getting sick from salmonella bacteria.

I find it amusing that many people think it's healthier to discard the yolk and only eat the white portion (protein). They don't realize the yolk contains all the heart healthy nutrients, such as lecithin and vitamin E.

Like any other food, when it comes to choosing eggs there can be major differences based on production methods and feed. In general, the best eggs come from smaller family-type operations that sell locally or regionally rather than the giant factory farms. These brands are sold mostly through independently owned natural food stores, farmer's markets, and co-ops. Look for eggs that are free-range and organically produced.

Milk

We've all seen the milk moustaches and heard the phrase "It does a body good." But if we put aside the marketing campaigns, what do we know about cow's milk? Is it a healthy beverage? Proponents argue that milk's benefits include weight loss, stronger bones, improved heart health and cancer prevention. Opponents claim that it causes obesity and increases risk of those diseases.

First, we must consider milk's intended role in life. It is nature's first superfood.

Nature designed it for rapid growth in newborns by providing a concentration of calories and essential nutrients. In France, a country with a lower rate of heart disease than the U.S., parents stop feeding their kids milk when they reach four or five years of age. Kids are then acclimatized into adult life with no special "kids' meals." Often, the kids will get a little wine in water instead of milk.

With age, a considerable number of people will lose their ability to produce lactase, an enzyme necessary for proper digestion of lactose, a sugar in milk. Apparently, nature did not deem it necessary to continue to produce lactase once we are weaned. However, when people first began dairy farming about 9,000 years ago in Northern Europe a gene variation was introduced that maintains lactase production. (Those with blood type B are said to do better with dairy foods as their ancestors were animal herders.) Hence, the wide variation of lactose-intolerance among ethnic groups and races. Less than 10 percent of Caucasians and the majority of Asians and Africans have difficulty digesting lactose. For those who can't handle lactose, consuming unfermented dairy products causes gas, bloating, cramps, constipation or diarrhea. You can diagnose yourself by drinking a glass of skim milk on an empty stomach. If within a couple of hours you don't have any gastrointestinal symptoms, you probably aren't lactose-intolerant.

Lactose-intolerant individuals often can tolerate fermented dairy foods, such as yogurt, buttermilk, cheese and kefir. During the fermentation process changes occur in milk due to the action of beneficial bacteria. The result of the bacterial action is a product that has reduced lactose, better digestibility and therapeutic effects the milk otherwise would not have. A large body of evidence confirms that lactic bacteria found in cultured dairy products and probiotic supplements help to maintain a favorable microbial condition in the intestinal tract associated with optimal health. Including these products in the daily diet provides many benefits, such as minimal lactose-intolerance, better digestion and absorption of milk protein, control of intestinal pathogens, an immune-enhancing effect, control of diarrhea, alleviation of constipation, lowering of serum cholesterol levels and an antitumor effect.

Dairy protein is a common food allergen, one of the so-called big eight (wheat, gluten, soybean, dairy, egg, fish/shellfish and peanut). Foods that are not digested properly tend to be mucus-forming and cause allergic reactions.

There are certain individuals who can benefit from milk drinking. If children or adults are not receiving, or do not have access to, a well-rounded nutritious diet, milk might help to compensate by providing needed calcium, vitamin D and other essential nutrients. It is, after all, a complete meal. If I had to choose, I would rather see kids drinking milk than sweet sodas. Most pediatricians advise switching to lower fat milk (2%, 1% or skim) after age two.

Some people object to the way milk is produced. For example, synthetic bovine growth hormones (BGH) are commonly given to cows to ramp up their milk production. The Food and Drug Administration (FDA) concluded that milk from BGH-treated cows is no different than milk from untreated cows and requires no special labeling to inform the consumer of its usage. FDA admits, however, that cows injected with BGH could suffer increased udder infections (mastitis), severe reproductive problems, digestive disorders, foot and leg ailments and persistent sores and lacerations, which may lead to increased amounts of pus and bacteria in milk. Equally disturbing is that these conditions will require treatment with powerful antibiotics and other drugs, which leave residues in the milk.

There are significant differences between raw milk and pasteurized-homogenized milk. The Textbook of Dairy Chemistry classifies pasteurized-homogenized milk as "denatured." Raw milk is what nature provides. It is untampered with and nutritionally superior.

Homogenization is a mechanical process in which milk is put under tremendous pressure and forced through a screen that reduces the size of the fat globules. This prevents the cream from separating and rising to the surface of the milk, producing a more uniform (homogenous) consistency.

The reduction in the size of the fat particles permits them to be assimilated in a manner not intended by nature. Some experts theorize that homogenization of milk contributes to plaque accumulation in arteries.

Pasteurized milk is milk that has been cooked—heated to 140-158 degrees F. for thirty minutes to destroy bacteria. Pasteurization was imperative during a time when disease-causing bacteria were carried by raw milk produced under unsanitary conditions. It is unnecessary if a proper environment is maintained.

Scientific literature verifies that pasteurization robs milk of vitamins B and C and more than a dozen heat-sensitive enzymes that are crucial to proper utilization of milk in the body. Milk must be fortified with vitamin D in an attempt to compensate for the absence of phosphatase, an enzyme that assists in the utilization of phosphorous and calcium. Pasteurization also destroys a natural germicide that inhibits bacterial growth. This explains the ironic fact that raw milk produced under hygienic conditions will keep longer than pasteurized milk when both are exposed to room temperature.

Dairies that specialize in raw, certified and organic milk products claim to have superior quality standards. Raw milk products are supplied by certified dairies that operate under extremely stringent government regulations and a strict industry code. These dairies test their milk daily for the presence of bacteria. At conventional dairies, these same tests are performed once a month. Employees of certified dairies are also tested. They submit to physical examinations and requests for throat cultures and stool specimens to identify infections, which might be transmitted to the herd.

Prejudice against raw milk exists, however. State officials have issued warnings and recalls linking raw certified milk and products to *Salmonella* poisoning in individuals without reasonable proof. If an infected person is known to have consumed a raw milk product it is assumed that this was the source of the infection. In truth, *Salmonella* bacteria are found everywhere—on meat, poultry, cutting boards, utensils, pets and humans. One could isolate *Salmonella* anywhere one tested for it. *Salmonella* poisoning has also been traced to pasteurized milk.

All of these factors need to be weighed in order to make an educated decision about dairy products. Whether cow's milk is healthful or not depends on who's drinking it and how much. In the minds of many, the scientific research is not clear. After 10,000 years, it is still a controversial, unresolved issue.

Coconut Oil

With references found in ancient Hindu scriptures, coconut is one of the oldest food plants. In the tropics, it has long been a dietary staple. Lately, coconut has become tremendously popular and trendy among health enthusiasts. The brown, hairy coconut is actually the seed of the coconut palm tree fruit. The oil is high in saturated fat, making it extremely stable (resistant to rancidity) and ideal for light frying.

Although mostly saturated (solid) fat, about half of it consists of medium-chain fatty acids (MCTs), which are rapidly burned by the body for energy. Research has not linked coconut oil consumption to heart disease. Instead, it actually appears to have a salutary effect by boosting beneficial HDL cholesterol and lowering certain risk factors. In moderately overweight individuals, coconut oil has been shown to promote thermogenesis (heat production) and calorie expenditure. Coconut oil also contains antiviral, anti-bacterial, and antifungal properties. Coconut oil recently became popular as a brain enhancer as a result of a viral online video that claimed it could cure Alzheimer's disease (AD). It told the story of how coconut oil helped a man's symptoms. Coconut oil is a rich source of the fatty acid caprylic acid. A preparation composed of caprylic acid, called Ketasyn, was used in a 2005 pilot study on AD patients and was found to improve memory in 47 percent of subjects.[1,2]

The beneficial mechanism of coconut oil and MCTs for the brain is believed to be an increase in brain cell energy. The primary energy source of the brain is glucose (blood sugar). However, in AD, there is a deficit in utilization of glucose, most often due to insulin resistance. (AD is sometimes called "diabetes of the brain.") Fatty acids in coconut oil can be used by the brain as an alternate source of energy and thus might improve symptoms of AD.

Coconut oil can be taken right off the spoon or used as a spread or dip. Because its melting point is 75-76 °F, coconut oil can be used in both liquid and solid forms for cooking and baking. It replaces butter on a 1: 1 basis in any baking recipe. Extra virgin, unrefined coconut oil has a mild coconut taste and aroma. Refined coconut oil is more neutral tasting and has a higher smoke point than extra virgin, so it is a better choice for sautéing and stir-frying. **MCT oil** is a highly-absorbable liquid source of caprylic and capric fatty acids with a minimal amount of lauric acid compared to regular coconut oil. MCT oil is not recommended for frying.

Soyfoods

Soy, a common staple of vegetarian diets, has been touted by growers, processors and many nutritionists as a miracle food. But lately the pendulum has swung in the opposite direction. Many authorities now say that soy's health benefits have been overblown and that it can actually be detrimental to one's health.

Like many other highly controversial issues, the truth often lies somewhere in the middle. You might be familiar with the saying "One man's food is another man's poison." This seems to be the case with soy. First let's look at soy's benefits.

To help keep things in perspective, let's point out that we're talking about a bean here, and beans are an important part of many healthy traditional diets. Vegetarians like soy because it's complete protein containing all essential amino acids. The Chinese call it "the meat without the bones." Soy protein also has a government approved health claim that it helps to lower risk of heart disease when part of a low-fat, low-cholesterol diet. In addition, soy is a source of phytoestrogens, which if not consumed to excess, can help to balance one's own estrogen levels. In Chinese women who consume soyfoods from an early age, there is a lower risk of breast cancer. Most soy consumed by this Asian population is in the form of fermented soyfoods, such as miso. Fermentation is said to improve digestibility and negate soy's negative properties.

The flipside is that soy is a common food allergen, one of the so-called big 8, which includes wheat, gluten, dairy, eggs, fish/shellfish, peanut and tree nuts. In addition, soyfoods can suppress thyroid function in people who have hypothyroidism and are lacking iodine. In women with pre-existing estrogen-sensitive breast cancer, some doctors advise limiting or avoiding soyfoods altogether.

Some soy enthusiasts may be going overboard by having too many soyfoods in their diet, such as soymilk, soy protein and tofu. The bottom line is that for most people, one or two servings of soyfoods per day can contribute to good nutrition. However, others (for reasons mentioned) may need to restrict soy in their diet.

Fish

Many people avoid fish because they believe our oceans are polluted. While it is true that eating certain fish may expose us to dangerous levels of certain toxins, the same can be said about land crops. Many crops are heavily sprayed with chemical pesticides that can increase risk of cancer.

Some types of fish may contain high levels of toxic mercury, which may pose a significant health risk, especially to pregnant or nursing women and children. Although mercury occurs naturally in the environment, the primary source of mercury in fish is coal-burning power plants. Most of the chemical toxins found in fish and shellfish originate with industry. They are released into the air and water, eventually making their way into the oceans. In the oceans, small fish low on the food chain ingest the toxins, which are transferred to, and accumulate in, larger predators—a process known as *biomagnification*.

Mercury is a neurotoxin that can harm the brain and nervous system. According to the Centers for Disease Control and Prevention, the blood of one in twelve Americans exceeds the Environmental Protection Agency's "safe" level for mercury. The highest levels of mercury are generally found in shark, swordfish, king mackerel and tilefish. Fresh tuna (which comes from larger fish than canned tuna) can also be high in mercury. Canned tuna (especially chunk light) does not have nearly as much mercury as fresh tuna, such as that consumed at sushi bars. Fish with the least mercury are blue crab (mid-Atlantic), catfish (farmed), croaker (not white), flounder, salmon (farmed or wild), shrimp and trout (farmed). Fish sticks and fast-food sandwiches are commonly made from fish that are low in mercury.

Mercury levels in the body drop substantially within a year if you switch from high-mercury species to low-mercury species. Every fifty days, on average, we eliminate half the mercury in our system.

Seafood provides a wide range of disease-fighting nutrients, making fish a healthy, smart food choice. Seafood is a rich source of protein, heart-healthy omega-3 fatty acids, vitamins, minerals, the carotenoid astaxanthin and RNA (ribonucleic acid). Although most types of fish are low in fat, many contain heart-healthy oils rich in the omega-3 fatty acids EPA (eicosapentaenoic acid) and DHA (docosahexaenoic acid). Good sources of EPA and DHA are salmon, mackerel, herring, anchovy, sardines, sablefish and trout. Because omega-3s tend to be lacking in the modern diet (about 85 percent of Americans are deficient), much emphasis has been placed on consuming more linolenic acid as well as active EPA/DHA. Numerous studies have found that EPA/DHA reduces the risk of cardiovascular disease and Alzheimer's disease, lessens symptoms of rheumatoid arthritis, reduces symptoms of ulcerative colitis and Crohn's disease, improves kidney function in severe diabetes, assists in optimal eye and brain development in infants, and eases depression and bipolar disorder.[3]

Our modern diet of processed and nutritionally depleted foods is generally believed to be the main contributor to declining health. Regular seafood consumption can help offset this trend, but we must choose wisely.

Gluten

Ever since man shifted from hunter-gatherer to food cultivator, humans have been challenged with altered nutrition. For many individuals, this change has proven to be too drastic for their digestive tracts. Wheat has been called "the staff of life," but its prevalence in the modern diet may be why it's now a common food allergen. Food repetition is believed to contribute to the development of food allergies, along with other factors such as stress and poor integrity of the intestinal lining.

Food allergy or hypersensitivity occurs when the body perceives certain proteins as a threat. Reactions can occur in any part of the body, with symptoms ranging from mild (excessive mucus production, indigestion, hives, for example) to severe (eczema, arthritis, depression). It's estimated that 60 percent or more of the American population suffers from symptoms associated with food reactions.

For some people, wheat and certain other grains are particularly toxic. Gluten, a protein in wheat, rye, and barley, has been identified as the culprit in celiac disease, a lifelong disorder in people who are genetically susceptible. In these individuals, gluten damages the mucosal surface of the small intestine, causing abdominal cramping, gas, diarrhea, constipation, oily stools, unexplained anemia, and weight loss or weight gain with a large appetite. If untreated, celiac disease can be life-threatening since damage to the intestinal lining can interfere with nutrient absorption. Although celiac disease affects less than 1 percent of the U.S. population, many shoppers perceive the phrase "gluten-free" on packaged foods as more healthful.

Individuals who are sensitive to wheat or other foods (dairy, for example) usually experience an improvement in symptoms when they rotate these foods in their diet. In other words, the food is not eaten more than once every three days. However, for those who have been diagnosed with celiac disease, it's imperative that they follow a strict gluten-free diet. This can be quite a challenge, though, since gluten is often hidden in foods. Ingredients that may contain gluten are hydrolyzed vegetable protein, textured vegetable protein, hydrolyzed plant protein, malt, modified food starch, soy sauces that contain wheat, and other prohibited substances and natural flavorings.

If you suspect that wheat or other foods are causing discomfort, try eliminating them from your diet. For a positive ID, ask a doctor about food allergy blood testing.

Appendix 5

The Tonic Herbs

YIN TONICS

Bee/Flower Pollen

Bee pollen is plant pollen collected by bees. It is the male seed of flowers, which enables flowering plants to reproduce. Pollen is the basis of the food chain on the land masses of the earth and contains all nutrients necessary to create new life within the plant world. It is a source of all known nutrients including twenty-two amino acids, twenty-seven mineral salts, and assorted vitamins, carbohydrates, fatty acids, enzymes and hormones. Approximately 3 percent of pollen's makeup is unknown and has been described as its mysterious "life force."

Bee pollen is collected from bees entering a monitored hive. As they pass through, a wire mesh screen scrapes the pollen from their legs. Some manufacturers have devised methods to eliminate bees from the collection process. This product is simply called "flower pollen."

A Swedish flower pollen extract uses a process that removes the hard pollen husk that accounts for more than 50 percent of its weight. The process makes the nutrients more bioavailable and results in a virtually non-allergenic extract that can be assimilated directly into the bloodstream and utilized on a cellular level. Much of the clinical research on pollen was performed using flower pollen extract.

Pollen extract has been used to manage symptoms of prostatitis and benign prostatic hypertrophy (BPH) in Europe for more than thirty-five years, and it has been the subject of double-blind clinical studies. Patients who respond typically have reductions in urinary frequency and nighttime urination of around 70 percent, as well as significant reductions in their residual urine volume.[1,2] This is likely due to its anti-inflammatory action as well as its ability to help the bladder contract while simultaneously relaxing the urethra.

In Russian studies involving people who had lived beyond one hundred years, it was discovered that a large number of them had been bee keepers who consumed honey and bee pollen. European doctors have experimented with pollen as a medicinal agent and have found that it is a strong biological stimulant with regenerative properties for human cells.

Bone Broth (Gelatin)

One of the hottest trends among health enthusiasts is bone broth. The nutrient-rich liquid is highly touted as an elixir for the skeleton, joints, immune system, and general vigor. It is one of the most potent Yin-nourishing substances in Chinese medicine.

Broths are essential components of major cuisines of the world and provide the foundation for soups, stews, and sauces. Most broths are made by boiling meats and veggies for a couple of hours, mainly for their flavor. Bone broth, however, is made by boiling animal bones for as much as twenty-four hours to extract the nutrients.

Bone broth provides a concentration of nutrients indigenous to our own bones and connective tissue (skin, hair, nails, joints, ligaments, and digestive tract). Key nutrients include collagen, amino acids, glucosamine, chondroitin, and minerals, which the body is able to easily digest and assimilate. Regular consumption is said to help with weight management, beautify the skin, calm inflammation, support joints and ligaments, and heal the lining of the digestive tract.

One celebrity who has testified to the benefits of bone broth is basketball legend Kobe Bryant. After suffering a severe ankle sprain caused by landing on an opponent's foot, he was taken out of the game indefinitely. On the advice of the team's nutrition director, he started consuming bone broth. Amazingly, he missed only two games. Not surprising, bone broth is now a regular part of his diet.

Bone broth recipes usually call for chicken and/or beef bones along with onion, carrot, and celery, which are simmered for twelve hours or more on a stove top or in a slow cooker. If you don't have time to watch the pot, you can turn if off at night then resume cooking the next day. When done, the broth is strained to remove the solids, which are discarded. Though it requires a long cooking time, preparation is easy. To some, it might seem like a big effort, but many people are becoming disenchanted with convenience-based fast-food culture. Fast foods may be easy, but they don't truly nourish our bodies.

Brewer's/Nutritional Yeast

Yeast is one of the most concentrated foods known. It is a rich source of protein (about 50 percent), B vitamins, minerals, and trace minerals such as selenium and chromium. Yeast also contains a high amount of ribonucleic acid (RNA), the messenger that carries genetic information needed to produce new cells in the body.

Yeast is a by-product of the beer brewing industry. However, much of it is grown today specially for human consumption on beets or molasses, which produces a better tasting product. Using 100 pounds of sugar as a growing medium, yeast will produce 65 pounds of high-quality protein, whereas a steer would yield only 1.2 pounds of beef.

Baker's yeast is different from nutritional yeast in that it contains live yeast cells. These yeast cells require B vitamins to grow, so if you were to eat it raw, it could rob you of vitamins rather than contribute to your store. When used in baking, the heat kills the yeast but leaves its nutrients behind.

Brewer's yeast has been used in the diets of mental patients and those with cirrhosis of the liver. It is good for pregnant and lactating women and has been recommended as a supplemental food for the elderly since it is so nutritious and inexpensive.

There is a misconception that eating yeast will cause a yeast infection. Food yeast (*Saccharomyces cerevisiae*) is not the same yeast that infects the bowels and vaginal cavity (*Candida albicans*). Yeast, however, is a common food allergen and, as with many other foods, some people may need to avoid it if they do not tolerate it.

Yeast can be added to all foods to increase their nutritional value. For best digestion and to decrease the possibility of a food reaction, take the powder or flakes in plain water or diluted fruit juice on an empty stomach before meals.

Cereal Grasses (Barley, Wheat)

Barley grass is one of the most highly researched green foods. It all began in the 1960s when Yoshihide Hagiwara, a Japanese scientist, started looking for the ideal food. After examining

150 different green plants, he decided that young barley grass had what he considered the most balanced nutritional profile.

Young barley grass has a higher nutrient value than the grain it eventually becomes. It is a rich source of vitamins, minerals, fatty acids, amino acids, enzymes, carotenoids, flavonoids, chlorophyll, and other phytonutrients. Since a plant's important nutrients reside in its juice component and not in its insoluble fiber content, green barley juice is separated from the fiber by extraction and then spray-dried into powder form. Tablets and powders are also available.

In the 1930s, researchers demonstrated that barley grass contains nutritional factors critical for normal growth and development. They found that during summer when cows could graze on fresh green grasses, their milk was superior to milk produced during winter when they were fed only dried food. Both human and animal studies demonstrate that barley grass supports cellular functions, promotes growth and development, enhances metabolism, helps control inflammation, provides antioxidant protection against free radicals and toxins, and enhances immunity and possibly longevity.

Many detailed case histories of patients demonstrate dramatic improvements to their health while taking green barley. They report that barley grass increases energy levels; gives them better-looking skin, hair and nails; improves their digestion; and reduces the occurrence of illness—all indicators of superior nutrition.

Wheatgrass is the young wheat plant. As a concentrated source of vitamins, minerals, chlorophyll, and enzymes, it is one of the most widely used supplemental health foods. Drinking fresh wheatgrass juice is an exceptional way to increase dark green leafy vegetables in the diet. At this early stage of the plant's life, it is considered a vegetable rather than a grain. Fifteen pounds of wheatgrass is the equivalent of 350 pounds of choice vegetables.

Ann Wigmore introduced wheatgrass juice to America more than fifty years ago. In her books, Wigmore calls it an ideal food to nourish the body and rid it of toxins. Wheatgrass is especially important to anyone who suffers from pain or illness.

Juicing unlocks the nutrients in vegetables and fruits, concentrating them and making them more bioavailable to the cells of the body. A sixteen-by-sixteen-inch tray of wheatgrass yields about 15 to 22 ounces of juice, depending on its length. Start with one ounce of wheatgrass juice per day. A therapeutic program might include as much as two to three ounces. Tablets and powder are a good second choice to fresh wheatgrass juice.

Chlorella

Chlorella is a single-cell, freshwater alga that contains nearly every nutrient necessary to sustain life. It is the basis for the food chain in nature's aquatic ecosystems. For humans and animals, chlorella is a complete food providing an array of nutrients including protein, EFA, fiber, vitamins, minerals, and phytonutrients. In short, chlorella is a superfood ideal for supplementing the modern, unbalanced diet of highly processed, nutrient-deficient foods.

NASA once studied chlorella and considered it a food of the future because it is a powerhouse of nutrients. For example, it contains a full spectrum of carotenoids including beta-carotene, alpha carotene, lutein, lycopene, and astaxanthin. A Harvard study concluded that 6 milligrams of lutein per day can reduce the risk of age-related macular degeneration, a cause of blindness, by 43 percent[3]. Just one serving of chlorella contains nearly this amount.

Chlorella's name is derived from the word "chlorophyll" because it is nature's richest source of chlorophyll (with ten times more than spinach). Chlorophyll is the pigment that gives plants their deep green color. It is the green "blood" of plants, which is chemically similar to our own blood. Its molecular structure closely resembles hemin, the pigment that combines with protein to form hemoglobin. Chlorophyll has magnesium at its core, whereas blood contains iron, giving it a red color.

Chlorophyll is a marvelous detoxifying and healing phytonutrient. It acts like a "magnet" in drawing out toxins from the body. It is an internal deodorant that cleanses tissues and is soothing and healing to injured tissue.

Chlorella is also the highest food source of RNA, referred to as chlorella growth factor (CGF), which supports healthy cell growth and development. DNA (deoxyribonucleic acid) is the genetic code of living organisms and is a "blueprint" of how we are constructed and how we function. RNA is the messenger that transmits instructions from DNA, directing the process of cellular renewal, growth, and repair.

In 1971, immune system resistance to cold viruses was demonstrated in a group of approximately one thousand Japanese sailors. Half of the men received 2 grams of chlorella a day, the others none. At the end of a three-month voyage, the untreated sailors suffered 41 percent more colds than the chlorella-takers.[4]

Ulcers, gastritis, hemorrhoids, inflammatory bowel, and other digestive disorders may benefit from regular chlorella use. The key ingredients appear to be chlorella's fiber and high chlorophyll content, which assist in healing injured tissue, increasing peristalsis, and stimulating growth of beneficial bacteria.

Research demonstrates that chlorella significantly binds and increases excretion of toxins, including mercury, arsenic, and cadmium[5]. It has been shown to reduce dioxin in breast milk.[6] Dioxins are potent carcinogens and endocrine disrupters. The research suggests that chlorella may help to lessen the risk of hormone-sensitive cancers of the breast and prostate. For highest digestibility, chlorella should have a thin cell wall or be processed by pulverization.

Ginseng, American

Ginseng is a term used to describe both American ginseng (*Panax quinquefolium*) and the Asian variety (*Panax ginseng*). Both have similar properties, but the Chinese regard American ginseng as a cooling Yin tonic, and Asian ginseng as a warming Yang tonic. Thus, American ginseng is used as a summer tonic, while Asian ginseng is used as a winter tonic. People who have plenty of energy, a high metabolism, an aggressive nature, or ruddy complexions can take American ginseng without concern of over-heating.

Panax is derived from the word "panacea," which means a cure for all diseases and a source of longevity as well as physical strength and resistance. American ginseng is often used in China to tonify the lungs of people with dry coughs due to smoking or pollution. It is said to moisten and cool the lungs.

Prior to its discovery in the early seventeenth century, American ginseng had been used by American Indians for purposes similar to the use of Asian ginseng by the Chinese. It was among the five most important medicinal plants of the Seneca people.

In the last thirty years, American ginseng has been extensively studied. Like *Eleuthero* (formerly called Siberian ginseng), ginseng is an adaptogen. At least seven European clinical studies showed that standardized extracts decreased reaction time to visual and auditory stimuli; increased respiratory performance, alertness, power of concentration, and grasp of abstract concepts; and improved visual and motor coordination.[7] A study conducted by French researchers evaluated complaints of patients suffering from fatigue, being worn-out and tired, and feeling empty.[8] The double-blind, placebo-controlled study involved 232 patients between ages twenty-five and sixty. Patients were allowed to choose five items from a list of twenty to best describe how they felt and to describe their response to either the test substance or placebo. Using a scale to score the conditions, patients were evaluated at twenty-one and forty-two days following treatment. At the end of the study, those who took a ginseng-containing product showed significant improvement in the scoring system when compared to patients who received the placebo. Improvement included parameters related to fatigue, anxiety/nervousness, and poor concentration. Recent studies have focused on antiviral and metabolic effects, antioxidant activity, and effects on nervous and reproductive systems.

Most American ginseng is produced in Wisconsin and the Canadian provinces of Ontario and British Columbia. Asian ginseng is cultivated in China, Korea, and Japan.

Goji

Goji (*Lycium barbarum*) is highly regarded by the Chinese as a longevity herb. The berries have been used for centuries in traditional Chinese medicine to treat poor vision, anemia, inflammation, and cough. The popularity of goji products has rapidly grown over the last decade, especially among martial artists. Studies show it is calming when one is overexcited and stimulating when one is depressed. It is said that eating a handful a day of the dried berries will make you happy for the rest of the day.

Goji is praised as an anti-aging remedy and is said to be one of the recommended herbs of Li Chun Yun, a Chinese herbalist who died in 1933 purportedly at the age of 256. Many of the identified constituents in goji are supported by scientific evidence for anti-aging effects. These effects include antioxidant action, immune regulation, and DNA protection.

Goji berries boast an extremely high rating on the Oxygen Radical Absorbance Capacity (ORAC) scale, an indicator of antioxidant potency. They've been shown to boost human blood antioxidant activity by up to 57 percent. A 2004 study showed that goji berries inhibited the formation of free radicals by an incredible 82 percent, further confirming their outstanding antioxidant properties.[9]

Goji berries are one of the richest known food sources of carotenoids that protect vision, including beta-carotene and zeaxanthin. Nearly 75 percent of the carotenoids in goji berries occur as zeaxanthin and the rest as beta-carotene. The main function of zeaxanthin is to absorb blue light and protect the delicate retinal area of the eye. Goji is the primary vision tonic in Chinese herbalism.

Green Defense®

Green Defense® is a Yin green food powder from Jarrow Formulas that provides juice powders from barley grass, wheat grass, and green vegetables, plus spirulina and green tea. It is rich in phytonutrients that support the body's self-defense mechanisms, detoxify and nourish the body, and assist in total well-being. Green Defense® can be helpful for those who fall short of their daily quota for vegetables.

Ho Shou Wu

Ho shou wu (*Polygonum multiflorum*) is a potent Yin tonic that is said to promote a long and healthy life, boost physical energy, enhance learning and memory, and promote sexual virility and sperm production. It is also reputed to nourish hair, teeth, bones, ligaments, and tendons and to prevent or reverse premature graying of hair. It is recommended as a rejuvenating physical and mental tonic for older men and women. Along with ginseng and goji, ho shou wu was recommended by Li Chun Yun. In Asia, it is widely used by athletes and martial artists. The whole root has been shown to lower cholesterol levels, according to animal and human research, as well as to decrease hardening of the arteries, or atherosclerosis.[10, 11]

Kelp

Kelp is a highly nutritious marine sea vegetable. Sea vegetables, or sea greens as some prefer to call them, contain practically every nutrient necessary to sustain life. Ideally, one should eat both land and sea vegetables every day to get a full complement of essential minerals. Sea vegetables, such as kelp, are far more concentrated in minerals than land vegetables. Land vegetables are only as good as the soil they are grown in, and studies show that the mineral content of our soil has steadily been declining due to intensive farming and chemical fertilizers. Seaweed, on the other hand, grows in a mineral-rich environment.

Kelp contains almost every mineral and trace element required for human existence, including vitamins, amino acids, and fiber. Kelp is also a principle source of iodine, superior to iodized salt. Iodine is an essential nutrient necessary for thyroid function, which helps regulate metabolism. In fact, one of the hormones produced by the thyroid gland (thyroxine) is composed of 65 percent iodine. So, if you eat more kelp you'll increase the efficiency of your metabolism.

Kelp is recommended for weight management, detoxification, immunity, and beauty. Eating kelp or taking kelp supplements helps to release excess body fluid and thin mucous deposits, which afflict bodies overfed with meat, dairy, and rich foods. It purifies the blood by helping neutralize tissues that are too acidic because of all the processed foods in our modern diet.

Kelp has a wide array of medicinal uses, including as an anticoagulant, diuretic, and lymphatic cleanser. Before the advent of antifungal drugs, iodine, which is found in high amounts in kelp, was the standard medical treatment for *Candida* yeast infections. Many scientists speculate that seaweed is probably a protective factor in the lower incidence of breast cancer among Japanese women. Research has shown that the darker sea vegetables such as kelp, kombu, wakame and hijiki, can remove radioactive elements from the body. Eating sea vegetables or taking an iodine supplement provides a measure of protection from radiation poisoning because it blocks the uptake of radioactive iodine by the thyroid.

Reishi

Reishi is called the "mushroom of immortality" and has been consumed in China for two thousand years both as an anti-aging herb and to improve the capacity of the mind and memory. Reishi is said to be a supreme shen (spiritual) tonic that invokes peacefulness, strengthens nerves, and changes how we perceive life. Conditions associated with disturbed shen include excessive mental activity, heart palpitations, insomnia, and stress.

Science validates many of reishi's positive health effects, which are extremely broad. Studies support its use for various conditions that can be grouped under several bodily systems, including the cardiovascular system, immune system and respiratory system. Reishi has been approved in Japan for treating certain types of cancers and has been used safely and effectively in conjunction with drugs or radiation.

Reishi has double-direction activity, which means it improves functioning of the immune system whether it is deficient or overactive. It doesn't stimulate the immune system; rather, it regulates it. Therefore, reishi is considered an immune modulator.

Ganoderic acids in reishi inhibit histamine release (allergic reactions), improve oxygen utilization and endurance, support liver functions, and scavenge free radicals. In Tibet, Himalayan guides use reishi to help combat high-altitude sickness. Chinese mountain climbers, who took reishi before ascending mountains as high as seventeen thousand feet, experienced minimal reactions to the climbs.

A study found that reishi extracts compared favorably with prednisone, a common steroidal anti-inflammatory drug with potentially serious side effects.[12] Reishi had few, if any, negative side effects. Note: The anti-inflammatory constituents of reishi, called triterpenes, are fat-soluble. These ingredients are concentrated by alcohol extraction. So, use tablets/capsules or liquids that contain both hot-water and ethanol (alcohol) concentrated extracts in order to achieve the maximum range of beneficial constituents.

Reishi is an excellent choice as an anti-stress herb to ease tension. It has been used routinely by monks, sages, shamans, and spiritual seekers. Many people who take reishi regularly notice that it brings peacefulness, an effect that cannot be explained by science. Reishi mushroom is too tough and woody to eat, so, look for it as a supplement.

Royal Jelly

Royal jelly is a thick, milky substance manufactured by bees from honey and pollen. When royal jelly is fed to an ordinary female bee in the larva stage, she is transformed into a queen bee. The queen is extremely fertile and lays more than twice her weight in eggs daily. She lives five to eight years compared to workers who live only two to six months. In human terms, this would be the equivalent of a person living to 1,320 years!

Scientists have been baffled by the queen's miraculous transformation. It is theorized that the queen's special food may actually be overriding DNA. Queens and workers have identical DNA, but the queen lives fifty times longer.

Royal jelly contains an array of nutrients, including B vitamins, minerals, enzymes, all eight essential amino acids, and, according to researchers at New York Medical College, the hormone testosterone, common to both men and women. Royal jelly is the richest source of pantothenic acid, which has been shown to increase the lifespan of animals. Royal jelly has similar applications as bee pollen and is believed to strengthen the reproductive system (men and women). Honey is often added to royal jelly to help preserve it. It is also available as pills.Shatavari Shatavari is a species of wild asparagus that grows in India and is the main Ayurvedic rejuvenative for women. It is commonly mentioned as a rasayana—an herb that promotes well-being by increasing vitality or resistance. Shatavari (*Asparagus racemosus*) means "she who possesses one hundred husbands," referring to its revitalizing effect on the female reproductive system. It is considered the female equivalent of ashwaganda, an herb frequently recommended as a male tonic.

Shatavari nourishes and cleanses the blood, and its healing qualities are useful in a wide array of conditions. Because it is a source of plant estrogens, it is a good choice for menopausal and postmenopausal women. In ancient Ayurvedic texts, it is specifically recommended in cases of danger of miscarriage and for stimulating the flow of milk in nursing mothers. Shatavari is an excellent aphrodisiac, improving sexual desire and enjoyment. Shatavari is used both as a single herb as well as a component of Ayurvedic herbal combinations for menstrual and menopausal support, blood sugar regulation, heart health, stress management, and geriatric care.

Shatavari is also useful for many conditions affecting the digestive tract. A study with rats showed that it protects against stomach ulcers induced by either stress or a pain medication (nonsteroidal, anti-inflammatory drugs).[13, 14] Researchers noted that shatavari significantly reduced gastric acidity while it increased levels of antioxidant enzymes and ascorbic acid. Its anti-ulcer effect was comparable to ranitidine, a standard anti-ulcer drug.

In Ayurveda, shatavari belongs to a group of herbs called medhya rasayanas, referring to the mind and intellect. These herbs are said to enhance one's ability to learn, retain, and recall information.

Spirulina

Spirulina (*Arthrospira platensis*) is a freshwater, single-celled alga that grows wild in lakes and is cultivated in ponds. Spirulina means "little spiral" and describes the plant's appearance under a microscope. This tiny plant is the basis for the food chain, supplying all nutrients necessary to sustain life within the water environment. Scientists define it as a simple hydrocarbon made directly from photosynthesis, the interaction of sunlight and water. One early spirulina researcher called it "imprisoned light."

Blue-green algae such as spirulina were the first life-forms to appear on the planet 3.5 billion years ago, producing oxygen in our atmosphere and allowing higher life-forms to evolve. More than five centuries ago in Mexico, wild spirulina was used as a food by the Aztecs. In Central America, archeological studies reveal that the Mayans may have used artificially constructed ponds for spirulina cultivation. It has also been speculated that manna, the divine food of the wandering Israelites that appeared miraculously on rocks, may actually have been dried spirulina. Today, spirulina is used by many people who value it as a nutrient powerhouse.

Gram for gram, spirulina contains more iron than spinach, as much calcium as milk, more beta-carotene than carrots, and more protein than steak. It is composed of approximately 60 percent protein, and it supplies eighteen of the twenty-two known amino acids, including all of the eight essential amino acids in balanced proportion. This makes spirulina a complete, high-quality vegetable protein.

Spirulina has vitamins in abundance. A 3 gram serving (about 1 teaspoon or six 500-milligram tablets) contains 6,000 units of beta-carotene—1,000 units more than the Recommended Daily Allowance (RDA) for beta-carotene (vitamin A). There are also generous amounts of B vitamins: One tablespoon contains 1.5 times more niacin and 307 times more potassium than a 1-cup serving of brown rice. Spirulina is especially notable for containing B12, the vitamin most difficult to obtain from vegetable sources. Beef liver was previously thought to be the richest source of this rare vitamin, but spirulina contains 250 percent more than beef liver.

The waters spirulina favors are so concentrated in minerals that no other microorganisms can grow there. Thriving in highly alkaline waters, the alga incorporates a large quantity of these minerals into its cell structure. Minerals that are organically bound to food are called chelated minerals, and unlike inorganic forms (obtained from rock or ore), they are easily assimilated by the body's tissues. Alkaline foods help to balance acidic foods like coffee, sugar, alcohol, and meat.

A unique feature of spirulina is its soft cell wall, which makes the nutrients highly bioavailable. Many plant foods have their nutrients locked up in tough, fibrous cell walls that require cooking or processing to make them accessible to the body's tissues. Spirulina, however, can be digested and absorbed with little effort, thus providing quick energy and nourishment. This is an important consideration for the elderly and undernourished who may not have efficient digestion and therefore, experience malabsorption.

The fat content of spirulina is low—between 4 and 7 percent—mostly in the form of the EFA linoleic acid and gamma linolenic acid (GLA). GLA is necessary to produce a family of local, short-lived hormone-like compounds called prostaglandins that control every organ in the body.

Microalgae are also loaded with chlorophyll. Chlorophyll is considered a cleansing and detoxifying phytonutrient that is also soothing and healing. Think of it as an internal deodorant that acts like a magnet, drawing toxins out of the body. Spirulina also contains a unique blue pigment called phycocyanin, which has both magnesium and iron at its center. Not surprisingly, spirulina has a beneficial effect on anemia, probably due to its blue-green pigments and bioavailable iron.

Spirulina is the most researched of all microalgae. Studies in the past years show that it is beneficial for many health concerns, including heart disease and obesity. Clinical trials suggest that taking several grams of spirulina daily can lower cholesterol. Other studies find a corresponding reduction in weight along with improved cholesterol levels. Taken before meals, spirulina seems to make a person feel more satisfied and less likely to crave sweets and desserts. Many food cravings are signals that the body is not sufficiently nourished.

Spirulina is an ideal supplement to take during a fast, since it sustains energy and assists the detoxification process without taxing digestion. It also supports bowel function by suppressing pathogenic bacteria and yeasts. Spirulina has obvious benefits for backpackers and athletes as well, and it is a good choice as a survival food.

Spirulina or Chlorella?

Spirulina and chlorella are freshwater algae that are highly touted as food supplements. I'm frequently asked how they differ and which is better. Spirulina is described as a photosynthetic bacterium whereas chlorella is a true plant with a cell nucleus. Both are excellent choices to augment or correct a deficient diet, especially one lacking in leafy green vegetables.

Spirulina is higher in beta-carotene and omega-6 GLA whereas chlorella would be the choice for nucleic acids (RNA/DNA), alpha-linolenic acid (omega-3), and B12. In Yin-Yang terms, chlorella is less cooling than spirulina. This property is beneficial to people who are attracted to warmth. Spirulina, on the other hand, might be the better choice for those attracted to cooler temperatures or with inflammatory conditions.

Tremella

Tremella fuciformis is popular in Asian cuisine and is one of the oldest cultivated mushrooms. Traditionally, the mushroom was consumed as a delicacy. Because it was rare, it was a luxury available only for the rich.

Also known as white jelly leaf, Tremella has a long history of use for nourishing the kidneys, lungs, and stomach and increasing moisture in the body. It is classified as a *Yin-jing* tonic, which means it enhances the primal energy of life by helping the body assimilate and store life-giving substances.

Some of the best health and beauty discoveries have come out of Asia, where techniques to achieve radiant health and beauty have been practiced for thousands of years. Yang Guifei, the courtesan of an eighth-century Chinese emperor, is said to be the most beautiful woman in Chinese history. She was so beautiful, in fact, she distracted the emperor from ruling, and the country began to fall apart. As the story goes, when she walked through a garden, the flowers bowed before her beauty. When asked what her beauty secret was she replied, "Tremella."

Tremella's skin-hydrating properties make it particularly useful as a beauty aid when taken internally or externally.

Proper hydration is the main objective of many popular cosmetic ingredients such as hyaluronic acid (HA). HA garnered much attention when it was discovered in the diets of long-lived inhabitants of a Yuzurihara, known as "the village of long life," outside of Tokyo. Here, degenerative diseases are rare, and few people show signs of aging in their skin. HA may deter aging by helping cells retain moisture, which keeps the skin smooth and elastic.

Cosmetic companies have recently begun to explore Tremella's promise as a cosmetic aid. When compared to HA, Tremella demonstrated a stronger water-holding capacity (five-hundred hundred times its weight) than sodium hyaluronate, a stable form of HA.[15] Tremella not only moisturized skin better but also helped the skin retain water longer. Tremella mushroom is now a key ingredient in a skin cream called Aquamella®. Tremella tablets and skin cream may be used together to maximize the benefits for nourishing skin, inside and out. In TCM, skin belongs to the lung network, and the lung provides proper moisturization to the skin. Tremella is said to remove facial freckles if used frequently.

Tremella is gelatinous and has a nearly white translucent color. The mushroom is composed of 70 percent fiber, which makes it useful for irregularity, weight management, and cholesterol control. Tremella contains the highest amount of vitamin D (ergosterol) among all edible natural foods.

YANG TONICS

Adrenal Optimizer®

Adrenal Optimizer® is a Yang tonic combination from Jarrow Formulas that contains *Rhodiola*, *Eleuthero*, ashwagandha, schizandra, and other supporting ingredients. It also provides shatavari, a Yin tonic. The adrenal glands produce hormones that underlie the body's mechanisms for coping with physical and mental stress. Factors such as overtraining in athletics and over-reliance on caffeine and other stimulants may tax the adrenals.

Ashwagandha

Ashwagandha is the Sanskrit word for *Withania somnifera*. Sometimes called Indian ginseng, it has a long use in Asia for strengthening one's constitution. The biochemical constituents found in ashwagandha appear to act as important regulators of hormonal processes in a balancing (adaptogenic) manner. When there is an excess of a certain hormone, ashwagandha constituents occupy receptor sites so that the effect of the hormone is muted. However, when the hormone level is low, ashwagandha constituents stimulate the receptor. The result is a balancing effect, which is particularly helpful for a healthy stress response.

When we encounter a stressful situation, the body automatically triggers the stress response. This involves the release of a number of signaling molecules from the adrenal glands that lie atop the kidneys. Epinephrine (adrenaline) and norepinepherine (the brain's version of adrenaline) initiate the "flight-or-flight" response. Glucocorticoids, such as cortisol, alter blood pressure, blood sugar, digestion, immune function, and even bone growth. This concerted response is meant to mobilize resources to increase the chances of survival in the present and avoid wasting energy for housekeeping and repair functions. This is an amazing survival response when we encounter occasional stressful situations.

However, if the stress response is constantly activated, the body runs into problems. Constantly elevated blood sugar levels can lead to changes in insulin sensitivity, while decreased housekeeping functions and a diminished immune response are problematic over the long-term. Unfortunately, this is what occurs with chronic stress. And this is why immune suppression, irregularities in glucose levels, elevated blood pressure, and other physiological effects are associated with chronic stress and, particularly, with chronically elevated levels of blood sugar-raising hormones. Ashwagandha appears to help modulate the activity of these messengers and temper their message.

Ashwagandha has been clinically shown to ease short-term stress, support normal levels of inflammation, promote a healthy outlook, support cognitive health, and increase physical endurance. In an animal study of rats exposed to mild, unpredictable footshock once daily for twenty-one days, those given ashwagandha one hour before better withstood the experience and responded with healthier blood sugar and sugar tolerance. They also experienced a normal range of corticosterone, healthy male sexual function, normal cognitive function, balanced immunity, and a healthy mood.[16]

In a placebo-controlled human study, participants experienced better mood scores, cortisol levels, C-reactive protein, and pulse rate and pressure, as well as normal levels of the adrenal hormone DHEA-S, hemoglobin, mean fasting blood sugar, and lipid profiles without unwanted effects.[17]

Recognized for centuries by practitioners of Ayurvedic medicine for its potent adaptogenic qualities, ashwagandha promotes physical and mental health and augments resistance against diverse environmental factors, revitalizing the body and supporting longevity.

It has been clinically shown to ease short-term stress, support the body's healthy inflammatory response, promote a healthy outlook, support cognitive health, and increase physical endurance.

Astragalus

Astragalus (*Astragalus membranaceous*) is one of the most widely used herbs in Chinese medicine. It has been traditionally known as the Great Protector. *Astragalus* in combination with ginseng is a well-known prescription in China. With ginseng, it is used as a tonic for fatigue, general debility, lack of appetite, and spontaneous perspiration.

Astragalus is becoming one of the better-known Chinese herbs for colds and as a general immune system stimulant. *Astragalus* is not a casual cold remedy. It is considered by most practitioners of Chinese medicine to be a deep immune tonic used to restore an immune system that is chronically stressed—for people who get one cold or flu after another and who believe that their defenses are down.

Asian researchers have extensively studied *Astragalus* because it is one of the important tonic herbs of traditional Chinese medicine. Pharmacological and clinical studies confirm its immunostimulant, antibacterial, antiviral, anti-inflammatory, adaptogenic, liver-protecting, and diuretic effects. It also improves stamina. Research shows that it protects white blood cells from destruction.

Cordyceps (Yin and Yang)

Cordyceps sinensis is a rare, potent, and highly treasured mushroom that was once used exclusively in the Chinese emperor's palace. It grows as a parasite on the larvae of a moth, mummifies the caterpillar, and sprouts the mushroom fruit off the caterpillar's head, before poking through the soil. More than 1,500 years ago, Chinese herders noticed that their animals became more energetic after eating these caterpillar mushrooms. Today, *Cordyceps* is commercially cultivated without the caterpillar.

Cordyceps strengthens lung power and is highly regarded in China as a tonic for those recovering from illness, an operation, or giving birth. In these instances, it helps patients recover physical energy while improving appetite and protecting the body from infection. In addition, *Cordyceps* contains various compounds that have anti-tumor and immunologic activities.

A group of Japanese researchers presented a paper showing that an aqueous *Cordyceps* extract dilated the aorta, the largest artery in the body, by 40 percent under stress. Dilation increases blood flow, which can benefit muscles that are pushed to their maximum, thus greatly enhancing endurance. The mushroom has general cardiotonic properties, which means it tends to increase the heart's muscle tone and inhibits cholesterol from being deposited in the aorta.

Cordyceps is a good choice for those who require energy for physical work. It is used by world-class athletes and has made international sports headlines. At the Chinese National Games in 1993, a team of nine Chinese women runners shattered nine world records, breaking the record for the 10,000-meter run by an unprecedented forty-two seconds. The athletes attributed their success to an intense training regimen and the use of *Cordyceps*.

Cordyceps is considered one of the best sexual tonics, although it is not quick acting. It is commonly recommended for frigidity, impotence, infertility, and sexual malaise. A clinical study of sexually dysfunctional men found that 64 percent improved in performance after ingesting one gram of *Cordyceps* per day.

Eleuthero

Eleutherococcus senticosus (formerly known as Siberian ginseng) is said to provide energy, endurance and an ability to withstand a wide range of adverse physical conditions. The use of Eleuthero in Chinese medicine dates back two thousand years. It was believed to provide energy and vitality and was used to prevent respiratory tract infections, colds, and flu.

Eleuthero is known as the "king of adaptogens" and has been the subject of more than three thousand studies. It is classified as an adaptogen because it helps individuals adapt to various types of stress and has a normalizing effect on a wide range of physiological imbalances. Eleuthero is believed to support adrenal gland function when the body is challenged by stress. Russian cosmonauts took Eleuthero to help them adapt to the rigors of spaceflight. After the Chernobyl nuclear accident in 1986, many Russian and Ukrainian citizens were given Eleuthero to counteract the effects of radiation. Studies show that the herb may enhance sensorial perception and heighten auditory awareness while protecting the hearing apparatus from damage due to excess stimulation. In addition, Eleuthero improves oxygen uptake by exercising muscles, enabling longer workouts and quicker recovery time for performance athletes.[18] It is said to be the safest and most healthful stimulant. Eleuthero is a good choice for both men and women and anyone seeking more energy for physical and mental activities.

Epimedium (Horny Goat Weed)

Epimedium is a very powerful Yang tonic. Loosely translated, the Chinese name means "the herb for the man that likes sex too much, like a goat." In general, this is what Epimedium is famous for and the most common purpose for using it.[19] It is relaxing yet sexually invigorating. The mechanism of Epimedium is similar to that of Viagra®, which enhances and relaxes smooth muscles by way of nitric oxide production.[20] In fact, the historical use of Epimedium in Chinese medicine was cited in the patent application for Viagra® to support the drug's claim for treating erectile dysfunction.

Ginseng, Asian

Ginseng (*Panax ginseng*) has been widely used as a folk medicine in China, Korea, and Japan for thousands of years, mainly as a general tonic and adaptogen to maintain the body's resistance to adverse factors, including improving physical and sexual function, general vitality, and anti-aging. *Panax* is derived from the word "panacea," which means a cure for all diseases and a source of longevity as well as physical strength and resistance. The German scientist Carl Anton Meyer thought ginseng was a cure-all, so he added the Latin name *Panax* in 1842. The Chinese, on the other hand, have never referred to it as a panacea, revered as it is. They named it ren-shen, which means "man root" because it has the shape of the human body. According to the Doctrine of Signatures, this tells herbalists that ginseng can be used to benefit the whole body. Ginseng is one of the most important tonics, crucial in addressing weakened energy states associated with aging, weakness following prolonged illness, and constant stress. The pharmacological effects of **ginseng** have been used for promoting immune function, improving central nervous system (CNS) function, relieving stress, and for its antioxidant activities.

Maca

Maca (*Lepidium peruvianum*) is a cruciferous vegetable (like broccoli) used by Peruvians as food and medicine. The root is highly prized for its powerful energizing and hormone-balancing effects. It grows up to fourteen thousand feet above sea level, making it the highest growing food plant in the world. Maca's cultivation goes back perhaps five thousand years. The Incas so prized the maca root that they restricted its use to their royal court. Conquering Spaniards soon became aware of the plant's value and collected tribute in maca roots to increase fertility in their animals.

A number of US medical doctors consider maca their herb of choice for reversing PMS, controlling menopausal symptoms, and weaning patients off hormone replacement therapy.

Although other natural remedies for menopause exist, such as black cohosh, dong quai, and soy isoflavones, maca works in an entirely different way from phytoestrogens and other herbal products, often with more satisfactory results. This is because it contains synergistic compounds that help the body make its own hormones rather than adding a weak plant hormone. Doctors have found that it greatly reduces or eliminates hot flashes, supports libido, increases vaginal lubrication, alleviates mood swings, and eliminates fatigue due to hormone imbalances.

Men, too, find that maca will counteract the difficulties they may experience in maintaining good sexual relationships as they age due to a slowing down of endocrine gland function. Because it helps maintain healthy levels of testosterone and DHEA, it is becoming popular with body builders, martial artists, and professional athletes who take it one hour before sports activity.

Maca is not recommended for people with a hormone-dependent cancer since it has not been specifically tested under these conditions. There are no known contraindications for maca, but allergic reactions have been reported by some (less than 1 percent). Since maca may unstick platelets and thin the blood, it is prudent to discontinue before surgery.

Rhodiola

Rhodiola rosea grows in the high-altitude polar regions of Europe and Asia. Rhodiola is believed to be the "Golden Root" of ancient legend. Its potential for improving physical and mental performance is unmatched.

Rhodiola is an adaptogen used for decades by Russian Olympians to maximize endurance and peak physical performance. Test subjects taking Rhodiola demonstrated greater back muscle strength and hand endurance, better coordination, and a more economical expenditure of oxygen. Any substance that is able to increase blood oxygen will provide a major advantage in terms of stamina and recovery.

In most Scandinavian countries, Rhodiola has been used for decades by professional athletes as a safe, effective, nonsteroid supplement to maximize endurance and accelerate muscular recovery[21]. Rhodiola extract has been shown to increase physical and mental performance by more efficiently mobilizing and sustaining muscular energy reserves.

There are three main physical benefits of Rhodiola that have been verified by more than one hundred research studies: It enhances muscle energy stamina during periods of peak physical stress; it speeds cardiovascular and muscle energy recovery time; and it possesses pharmacologically relevant anabolic activity.

Schizandra

Chinese women have historically held schizandra in high esteem because of its beauty-enhancing qualities. It is said to protect the skin from the damaging effects of the sun and wind. If used for a hundred days, it is said to make the skin radiantly beautiful. Schizandra possesses all five tastes (sweet, sour, salty, bitter, and pungent). Its Chinese name is *wu wei zi*, which means "five-taste fruit." Schizandra is used by both men and women for sexual vigor and to promote secretion of sexual fluids (semen and vaginal secretions). Schizandra is considered a mind tonic that improves memory and sharpens focus.[22] Schizandra supports liver function and detoxification and antagonizes the stimulating effect of caffeine.[23]

Resources

Mushroom Wisdom

www.MushroomWisdom.com

Mushroom Wisdom, located in East Rutherford, New Jersey, is a global leader in the development, production, and research of mushroom supplements. Products include Maitake D-Fraction®, SX-Fraction®, Amyloban® 3399, *Cordyceps*, lion's mane, shiitake, double-extraction reishi, *Tremella*, and paraben-free Aquamella® skin cream. The mushroom supplements are hot-water extracted from the fruiting body, with the exception of *Cordyceps*. Growth medium is native substrate (oak and birch), not grain. Use tablets, capsules, or liquids that contain both hot-water- and ethanol- (alcohol) concentrated extracts from the mushroom fruiting body, not mycelium, in order to achieve the maximum range of beneficial constituents.

Jarrow Formulas

www.Jarrow.com

Jarrow Formulas, based in Los Angeles, California, is a formulator and supplier of superior nutritional supplements. The company markets its products in the United States, Mexico, and Canada, and throughout the world. Products include Whey protein, Organic Flaxseed Oil, Coconut Oil, MCT Oil, Green Defense®, and Adrenal Optimizer®. Green Defense® is a Yin tonic that provides juice powders from barley grass, wheat grass, and green vegetables plus spirulina and green tea. Adrenal Optimizer® is a Yang tonic that contains *Rhodiola*, *Eleuthero*, ashwagandha, schizandra, and other supporting ingredients.

Ken Babal Nutrition Counseling

www.NutritionMusician.com

The author is a health practitioner who offers personalized nutrition programs for health enhancement. Services include weight management (adults and kids), cardiovascular, immune and digestive health, anti-aging strategies, stress management, blood sugar control, detoxification programs, and sports nutrition.

National Certification Commission for Acupuncture and Oriental Medicine (NCCAOM)

www.nccaom.org

A national, non-profit organization and referral source for oriental medicine practitioners, acupuncturists, and Chinese herbologists.

Notes

Chapter 1: The Yin-Yang Concept

1. Herman Aihara. *Acid and Alkaline*. (George Ohsawa Macrobiotic Foundation, 3rd ed., 1980).

Chapter 2: Protein and Essential Fatty Acids

1. Udo Erasmus, *Fats That Heal, Fats That Kill* (Alive Books, 1993).
2. Will Brink, *Life Extension Magazine* (September 2013): 51-63.

Chapter 3: Fats and Oils

1. Paul Pitchford, *Healing with Whole Foods: Asian Traditions and Modern Nutrition* (North Atlantic Books, 2002).
2. Ken Babal, CN, *Seafood Sense: The Truth about Seafood Nutrition and Safety* (Basic Health Publications, 2005).
3. M.C. Morris et al. "Consumption of fish and n-3 fatty acids and risk of incident Alzheimer's disease." *Arch Neurol*, no. 60 (2003): 940-946.
4. M de Lorgeril et al. "Mediterranean alpha-linolenic acid-rich diet in secondary prevention of coronary heart disease." *Lancet* 343 (1994): 1454-9.

Chapter 4: Carbohydrates: Refined and Unrefined

1. Barry Sears, *The Zone* (Harper Collins, 1995), 30.
2. Ken Babal and Mark Kaylor, *Syndrome X and SX-Fraction* (Woodland Publishing, 2003).
3. Argiles JM, Lopez-Soriano FJ. "Insulin and cancer (review)." *International Journal of Oncology* 18 (2001): 683-87.
4. S. M. De la Monte and J.R. Wands. "Alzheimer's Disease is Type 3 Diabetes-Evidence Reviewed." *Journal of Diabetes Science Technology*, 2 no. 6 (November 2008): 1101-1113.
5. Michael Stern. "Insulin Signaling and Autism." *Frontiers in Endocrinology* 2 (2011): doi:10.3389/fendo.2011.00054.

Chapter 5: Sodium and Potassium

1. Herb Boynton, *The Salt Solution* (Avery, 2001).
2. Dr. Richard Moore interviewed by Richard A. Passwater, PhD. "Potassium-to-Sodium Ratio Affects Overall Health, Part 2: Imbalance Often Leads to Hypertension." *Whole Foods Magazine* (June 2001, 54-60.).

Chapter 6: Digestion and Elimination

1. Ken Babal, CN, *Good Digestion: Your Key to Vibrant Health* (Alive Books, 2000).
2. Zosia Chustecka "Dramatic 50% Rise in Esophageal Cancer in British Men." *Medscape* https://www.medscape.com/viewarticle/729241 (Sep 22, 2010).
3. Willy Gomm, PhD, Association of Proton Pump Inhibitors With Risk of Dementia, *JAMA Neurology* 73 (2016): 410
4. Zhou B, Proton-pump inhibitors and risk of fractures: an update meta-analysis.*Osteoporosis International* 27 (2016): 339.
5. Jonathan V. Wright and Lane Lenard, *Why Stomach Acid is Good for You* (M. Evans and Company, Inc., 2001).

Chapter 7: Food and Food Abstinence

1. Roy Walford, *Maximum Life Span* (Norton, 1983).
2. Ibid.
3. M. Harvie et al. "The effects of intermittent or continuous energy restriction on weight loss and metabolic disease risk markers: a randomized trial in young overweight women." *International Journal of Obesity* 35 (2011): 714.
4. M. Harvie, et al. "The effect of intermittent energy and carbohydrate restriction v. daily energy restriction on weight loss and metabolic disease risk markers in overweight women." *British Journal of Nutrition* 110 (2013): 1534.

Chapter 8: Acid and Alkaline

1. Sigrid Jehle et al. "Effect of potassium citrate on bone density, microarchitecture, and fracture risk in healthy older adults without osteoporosis: a randomized controlled trial." *Journal of Clinical Endocrinology and Metabolism* (November 15, 2002): jc2012-3099.

2. M. Kendall et al. "Potassium citrate supplementation results in sustained improvement in calcium balance in older men and women." *Journal of Bone Mineral Resources*. (February 15, 2013): 1764.: doi:10.1002/JBMR.

3. T.R. Remer et al. "Estimation of the renal net acid excretion by adults consuming diets containing variable amounts of protein." *American Journal of Clinical Nutrition* 59 no. 6 (1994): 1356-1361.

4. Durk Pearson and Sandy Shaw, *Life Extension: A Practical and Scientific Approach* (Warner Books, 1982): 249.

5. G. Schwalfenberg. "The Alkaline Diet: Is There Evidence That an Alkaline pH Diet Benefits Health?" *Journal of Environmental Public Health* https://www.ncbi.nlm.nih.gov/pmc/articles/PMC3195546/ (2012).

Chapter 9: Basic Meal Planning

1. Penn State. "Penn State Diet Studies: To Weigh Less, Eat More." ScienceDaily. ScienceDaily, 1 December 2004. <www.sciencedaily.com/releases/2004/11/041123204013.htm>.

2. E. Giovannucci et al. "A prospective study of tomato products, lycopene, and prostate cancer risk." *Journal of the National Cancer Institute* 94 (2002): 391-8.

Chapter 11: Yin Tonics and Yang Tonics

1. Daniel B. Mowrey, Ph.D. Herbal Tonic Therapies (Keats Publishing, 1993).

Appendix 1: Beverages

1. H. F. Stich, "Teas, and tea components as inhibitors of carcinogen formation in model systems and man." *Prevalent Medicine* 21 (1992): 377-384.

2. K. Nakachi et al. "Influence of Drinking Green Tea on Breast Cancer Malignancy Among Japanese Patients." *Japanese Journal of Cancer Research* 89 (1998): 254-261.

3. S. Gupta et al. "Prostate Cancer Chemoprevention by Green Tea." *Seminar of Urology Oncology* 17 (1999): 70-76.

4. A. G. Dulloo et al. "Efficacy of a green tea extract rich in catechin polyphenols and caffeine in increasing 24-h energy expenditure and fat oxidation in humans." *American Journal of Clinical Nutrition* 70 (1999):1040-1045.

5. Dallas Clouatre. "Green Mate for Energy, Weight Control and More." *Total Health Magazine* 26.1.

6. James D. Lane et al. "Caffeine Affects Cardiovascular and Neuroendocrine Activation at Work and Home." *Psychosomatic Medicine* 64 no. 4 (July-August 2002): 595-603.

7. "Alcohol: Balancing Risks and Benefits," Harvard TH Chan School of Public Health, accessed August 22, 2018, www.hsph.harvard.edu/nutritionsource/healthy-drinks/drinks-to-consume-in-moderation/alcohol-full-story/.

Appendix 2: Sweeteners

1. K. Watanabe et al. "Anti-influenza viral effects of honey in vitro: potent high activity of manuka honey." *Archives of Medical Research.* 45 no. 5 (May 29, 2014): 359-65. doi:10.1016/j.arcmed.2014.05.006. Erratum in: *Arch Med Res.*45 no. 6 (August 2014): 516.

2. S. B. Almasaudi et al. "Antioxidant, Anti-inflammatory, and Antiulcer Potential of Manuka Honey against Gastric Ulcer in Rats." *Oxidative Medicine and Cell Longevity* (December 7, 2015): 3643824. doi: 10.1155/2016/3643824.

3. S. Anton et al. "Effects of stevia, aspartame, and sucrose on food intake, satiety, and postprandial glucose and insulin levels." *Appetite*, 55 no. 1, (August 2010): 37-43.

Appendix 4: Food Facts and Fallacies

1. Ketasyn in Mild to Moderate Alzheimer's Disease. https://clinicaltrials.gov/ct2/show/NCT00142805

2. Michael Murray, "The Health Benefits of Coconut Oil," *Vitamin Retailer*, May 2018, 54-56.

3. Ken Babal, CN. *Seafood Sense: The Truth About Seafood Nutrition and Safety*, Basic Health Publications (2005), p. 20.

Appendix 5: The Tonic Herbs

1. A. C. Buck et al. "Treatment of outflow tract obstruction due to benign prostatic hyperplasia with the pollen extract, Cernilton. A double-blind, placebo-controlled study." *British Journal of Urology* 66 no. 4 (1990): 398-404.

2. S. Dutkrewicz. "Usefulness of Cernilton in the treatment of benign prostatic hyperplasia." *International Urology and Nephrology* 28 no. 1 (1996): 49-53.

3. Johanna M. Seddon et al. "Dietary Carotenoids, Vitamins A, C, and E, and Advanced Age-Related Macular Degeneration." *Journal of American Medical Association* 272 (1994):1413-20.

4. Y. Kashiwa and Y. Tanaka. "Effect of Chlorella on the changes in the body weight and the rate of catching cold of the 1966 training fleet crew." Japan Medical Science Meeting (Nagoya, Japan, 1966).

5. Jae-Young Shim et al. "Protective Effects of *Chlorella vulgaris* on Liver Toxicity in Cadmium-Administered Rats." *Journal of Medicinal Food* 11.3 479-85 (September 18, 2008).

6. Shiro Nakano, et al. "*Chlorella* (*Chlorella pyrenoidosa*) Supplementation Decreases Dioxin and Increases Immunoglobulin A Concentrations in Breast Milk." *Journal of Medicinal Food* 10 no. 1 (May 1, 2007) 134-142.

7. "Ginseng," Stephen Foster Group, accessed August 22, 2018, www.stevenfoster.com/education/monograph/ginseng.html.

8. M. Le Gal et al. "Pharmaton Capsules in the Treatment of Functional Fatigue: A Double-blind Study Versus Placebo Evaluated by a New Methodology." *Phytotherapy Research* 10 no. 1 (1996): 49-53.

9. S.J. Wu et al. "Antioxidant activities of some common ingredients of traditional chinese medicine, *Angelica sinensis*, *Lycium barbarum* and *Poria cocos*." *Phytotherapy Research*. 18 no. 12 (December 20014):1008-1012.

10. S. Foster and Y. Chongxi. *Herbal Emissaries: Bringing Chinese Herbs to the West*. (Rochester, VT: Healing Arts Press, 1992): 79-85.

11. S. Foster, *Herbal Renaissance*. (Layton, Utah: Gibbs Smith, 1993): 40-41.

12. Ming-Chun Wen et al. "Efficacy and tolerability of antiasthma herbal medicine intervention in adult patients with moderate-severe allergic asthma." *American Academy of Allergy, Asthma and Immunology* (2005) 517-524.

13. M. Bhatnagar et al. "Antiulcer and antioxidant activity of Asparagus racemosus Willd and Withania somnifera Dunal in rats." *Annals of the New York Academy of Sciences.* 1056: (November 2005): 261-78.

14. Bhatnagar et al. "Antisecretory and antiulcer activity of Asparagus racemosus Willd. against indomethacin plus phyloric litigation-induced activity gastric ulcer in rats." *Journal of Herbal Pharmacotherapy* 6 no. 1 (2006): 13-20.

15. Yukihiro Ohashi and Yasuko Yamamoto. "Mechanisms of polysaccharide and their application to the cosmetics: Tremella fuciformis polysaccharide." *Fragrance Journal* (2005).
16. Bhattacharya et al. "Adaptogenic activity of Withania somnifera: an experimental study using a rat model of chronic stress." *Pharmacology, Biochemistry and Behavior* 75 (2003): 547–555.
17. Biswajit Auddy et al. "A Standardized Withania Somnifera Extract Significantly Reduces Stress-Related Parameters in Chronically Stressed Humans: A Double-Blind, Randomized, Placebo-Controlled Study." *Journal of American Nutraceutical Association* 11 (2008): 50-56.
18. GS Kelly, Sports nutrition: A review of selected nutritional supplements for endurance athletes," Alternative Medicine Review 2 no. 4 (1997): 282-95.
19. Ron Teeguarden, *Radiant Health: The Ancient Wisdom of the Chinese Tonic Herbs* (Warner Books, 1998).
20. J. H. Chiu. "*Epimedium brevicornum* Maxim extract relaxes rabbit corpus cavernosum through multitargets on nitric oxide/cyclic guanosine monophosphate signaling pathway." *International Journal of Impotence Research* 18: (2006): 335-342.
21. R. D. Seifulla, *Sport Pharmacology Manual* (Sport Pharm Publishing: Moscow, 1999): 104.
22. Teeguarden *Radiant Health*: 147
23. Ed Smith, *Therapeutic Herb Manual: A Guide to the Safe and Effective Use of Liquid Herbal Extracts* (Ed Smith Publisher, 2011): 63.

Index

About the Author

Ken Babal has a clinical nutrition practice in Los Angeles and is a consultant to the natural food and dietary supplement industry. He has written more than five hundred articles that have appeared in many popular and professional publications and is author of several books, including *Mushrooms for Health and Longevity* (Alive Books, 2011), *Seafood Sense: The Truth about Seafood Nutrition and Safety* (Basic Health Publications, 2005) and *Good Digestion: Your Key to Vibrant Health* (Alive Books, 2000). He appears in the Discovery Health Channel documentary "Alternatives Uncovered," and E! TV's "The High Price of Fame: Starved!" Ken is a frequent guest on radio and TV and presents seminars at stores and industry events across the country. Visit his website at www.NutritionMusician.com.